IS A HOME BIRTH RIGHT FOR YOU?

EVIE STEINHART, RN

ISBN 978-1-7360609-1-9 (ebook)
ISBN 978-1-7360609-0-2 (print)

Library of Congress Control Number: 2020922712

To contact author/publisher

email ihomebirthmom@gmail.com

DEDICATION

To my husband with deep gratitude.
I couldn't have done it without you.

ACKNOWLEDGEMENTS

"It is good to give thanks to God and to sing His Name on high. To tell in the morning of His kindness and in the evening of His faithfulness."
Psalms (92:2,3)

Thank you to the following people for your contributions to this book: Pearl Steinhart, Leah Marinelli, Lauren Bildner, Natasja Eby, Joanne Machin, Shira Kosowsky, Mary Cain, Samantha Elphick, Jennifer Griffin, April Davis, Tara Rose, Jessica Cole, Chaya Jacobs, Yehudit Debrova, Renske Kuiper, Ruthie Pearlman, Sarah Lewis, Hannah Dahlen, Eugene DeClercq, Asifat Kunle Lukeman, Ank De Jonge, Tamar Van Haaren-Ten Haken, Helen Robinson, Anne Cobell, Yetty Engel, Carina Primavesi, Hammad Khalid, Batsheva Nagel, Shoshana Levy, Debi Brunt, Barbara Ben Ami, and Mindy Levy.

Thank you to my husband and kids for encouraging and supporting me.

And finally, thank you to my Mum for showing me what a strong woman looks like, and for raising me with the belief that I can do anything I put my mind to.

"The home birth experience is intimate, empowering, beautiful, transformative. For someone who is inclined to do it, it is a very special thing to do. Home birth teaches you a lot about your body's wisdom and about family strength. It's just a really beautiful experience."
~Lauren Bildner, CNM

Contents

Foreword

By Dr. Judith Lothian PhD, RN, FAAN

When I had my first baby, almost all women gave birth alone in a haze of "twilight sleep". Although they felt every contraction they remembered nothing and asked for hours after the birth of their baby "What did I have?" I wanted something different. I wanted my husband with me and I didn't want "twilight sleep." I was a nurse and as a student I had the good fortune to be with just one woman who gave birth "naturally." It changed my thinking about birth. I went on to have a natural birth years later and that birth transformed me.

My transformation was both personal and professional. Becoming a mother is meant to be a transformative experience. The experience also changed the direction of my nursing. I became a childbirth educator and eventually a nursing professor teaching, writing and doing research about birth and breastfeeding. In the last decade the focus of my research has been on women's and midwives' experiences of home birth.

My last baby was born 18 years after my first baby. How the world of birth had changed! In 1969 the cesarean rate was 6%. By 1987 it was on the rise. Today it hovers around 31%. Maternal mortality rates had not yet started to rise but today the rate is the highest in the developed world. Routine interventions, like restrictions on eating and drinking, intravenous fluids, continuous electronic monitoring, and restrictions of movement had become the norm.

While we had learned a lot about ways to find comfort in labor, in too many hospitals the epidural was then and continues to be the only comfort option available for women in labor. In many ways it has become more difficult to have that natural birth.

While hospital birth continues to be "intervention intensive" even for healthy women with no medical complications, women today have many more choices than I had for any of my births. Midwives are once again an important part of the maternity care system. And women in an increasing number of places have the option of giving birth outside the hospital in either a birthing center or in their own home. The availability of these options is driven by a deeper understanding of the physiology of labor and birth and an increasing body of research that supports the value and importance of allowing that process to unfold without interference. Interfering in the physiologic process of birth without true medical indication actually increases risk for mother and baby. And the increase in options is also driven by many women wanting to avoid the intervention intensive labor and birth on offer in hospitals. In fact, in my own research on home birth, I interviewed[1] women about how they made the decision to give birth at home. The women I interviewed wanted to avoid unnecessary interventions; wanted to know their midwife and for her to know them, knowing they would feel comfortable and protected at home, and knowing that hospital medical care was available if needed.

I began to write about midwifery care and out of hospital birth as a way to decrease interventions, decrease the cesarean rate and increase women's satisfaction with childbirth. But I had never actually been at a home birth. That changed when my daughter Mary had her third baby at home after 2 birthing center births with a midwife. I was again transformed. I was struck with the calmness, the level of support, the absence of "stuff" like fetal monitors, intravenous, and restrictions of any kind. The midwife "caught" the baby rather than "deliver" her. Minutes after the birth with Baby Maggie skin to skin with her mother, the big sisters (2 and 4 years old) climbed on the bed with their Mama to meet their little sister. The midwife made tea and fed my daughter bits of fruit and cheese then helped her into the shower. I made a wonderful dinner and while mother and baby rested together our extended family celebrated Maggie's birth a few rooms away. Mary went on to have 3 more home births with the older children present at the births of the new babies.

The decision to give birth outside the hospital and/or with a midwife is an intensely personal one. It is also a decision that is best made with full information. Stunningly, while there is a great deal of research on the value and safety of midwifery care and home birth for healthy women with no pregnancy complications, there is still very little literature for women and their families who are thinking about home birth and want to know more.

This book helps fill that gap in the literature. You will learn about the history of birth, the physiology of birth, the criteria for a safe home birth…including being a healthy woman, having an experienced health care provider, and a plan for safe, quick transfer to a hospital if complications begin to develop. You will also learn some practical things…like choosing who will be with you at your birth, what supplies you need, what the midwife brings to the birth, the importance of support. And you will hear women's stories, perhaps the most valuable part of your reading.

You are fortunate to have choices. This book will, I hope, help you make your decision.

Dr. Judith Lothian, PhD, RN, FAAN

Graduate Chair at Seton Hall University College of Nursing

Associate Editor of the *Journal of Perinatal Education*

Author of *The Official Lamaze Guide: Giving Birth With Confidence*[2]

PREFACE

Ask any mother about the birth of their child and they will have a story to tell you. Birth is life-altering, a moment a woman never forgets. Women relate their birth stories throughout their lives and relive the wonder of that moment each and every time.

No matter what kind of birth experience a mother has, it is transformative. No one is guaranteed a perfect birth or the birth of their dreams, but you CAN shape your experience by the choices you make around who will deliver your baby, who will accompany you during labor, and where you will give birth.

I hope this book will guide you in making the choices that are right for you and your family.

INTRODUCTION

For most home birth parents, the decision to have a home birth is not a quick and easy one. Most home birth parents think long and hard before deciding to have a home birth. For me, making the decision to have a home birth was the culmination of a process that started years before I actually had one.

My first introduction to natural birth came from my maternity instructor in nursing school. Her name was Mrs. Greenbaum and she was a strong believer in woman-centered care. During our semester together, she took our class down to the Elizabeth Seton Birthing Center in Lower Manhattan to show us what unmedicated natural birth can look like. It was a stark contrast to what women were experiencing in our maternity clinical rotations at the local hospital.

Several years later, I spent two years working on a maternity floor at a major New York hospital. There I saw how women were cared for by doctors, nurses, and midwives. I saw how they were spoken to, the choices they were offered, and how their birth experiences turned out.

When I was pregnant with my first child, I really wanted a home birth but my husband was not on board with the idea. We went to a local midwifery practice that delivered in a nearby hospital, and I hired a highly recommended doula. I had an amazing natural birth that could not have gone any better. The nurses at the hospital were supportive and encouraging and really worked as a team with my midwife and doula.

With my second baby, the hospital where I delivered my first child had closed down. I hired the same doula who had accompanied me to my first birth, but I delivered with a different midwife at a different hospital. I had a natural birth but did not love my experience. Unfortunately, this hospital had protocols in place that were unpleasant and unnecessary.

When I was pregnant with my third baby, I found a midwife who delivered both at home as well as at a local hospital. As my husband had serious reservations around the safety of having a home birth, my midwife sat with us one evening for about two hours listening to us and addressing our concerns. She discussed her safeguards, standards, and protocols for managing emergencies that may occur. We felt reassured that my safety and our baby's safety were paramount, and we went on to have a beautiful home birth.

My fourth baby was born at a local hospital, as our insurance had changed, and we had difficulty getting a home birth approved. The hospital had a birthing tub which was really nice, and the birth went well.

My fifth baby was born at a home birth, and my sixth child was born at home as well. As the COVID-19 pandemic was in full swing during my last home birth, I was very grateful I didn't have to go in to the hospital. Interestingly, I found friends and family much more accepting of our decision during that time. I'm hoping this will signal a change in the level of acceptance society directs at parents choosing to have a home birth.

If you've picked up this book, you probably have many questions about home birth. I think the primary question people have when considering a home birth is around its safety. Is a home birth as safe as delivering in the hospital?

Other questions that you may have include:

Why is home birth more accepted in some communities than others?

Why are there different standards of education among midwives in the United States and around the developed world?

Why are some midwives more strict with criteria for a home birth than other midwives?

Why are women increasingly turning to home births to avoid going to the hospital?

While writing this book, I interviewed birth professionals and home birth moms from around the world to obtain answers to these questions. The interviews were incredibly insightful and informative, and I included many passages from the interviews in this book. You can find the interviews in full on my website www. homebirthmom.com.

In addition to the interviews, a lot of research studies are cited in this book. This is done in order to back up information with hard data and statistics so that you can draw your own conclusions on the significance of the studies.

I hope you find answers to your questions in this book, and I hope this book will give you the tools you need to choose the right setting for you and your baby.

CHAPTER 1

Why a Home Birth?

Most people consider their home a place of comfort. It is our refuge, one we share with our nearest and dearest.

Our values and beliefs are reflected in the pictures and artwork adorning our walls, in the style and configurations of our furniture and décor. It is our own intimate and sacred space, a place where we can just be ourselves. The simple truth is that moms will labor best in a place where they feel safe and protected.

Think about it for a moment: Your physical state mirrors your emotional state. When you are anxious, your muscles tighten, your jaw clenches, and your breathing becomes shallow. In contrast, when your mind is calm, muscle tension dissipates, and your body relaxes.

The process of labor is regulated by the mother's nervous system. For labor to begin and progress, the body releases the hormone oxytocin in increasingly greater amounts. This, in turn, increases the strength and duration of your contractions, driving your labor forward. Oxytocin is also known as a "love hormone," as it is released when you are feeling loved and cared for. On the other hand, tensing up and feeling stressed complicates labor and prolongs[3] it. As such, childbirth educators agree that relaxing the mind and body is central to an easy quick labor[4].

With this understanding in mind, home birth midwives endeavor to provide a calm and quiet environment during labor.

Hannah Dahlen[5], professor of midwifery at Western Sydney University in Sydney, Australia, and home birth midwife, describes the contrast between a hospital birth and a home birth experience in vivid detail:

> I think unless you've had a home birth, or been at a home birth, it's really hard for the general public to understand how different it is. Before I went in to do home births, I'd been a midwife for thirty years, and I had worked for twenty years in high-risk maternity units, most of the time in the delivery ward, so I was a very expert midwife. I could suture in the dark, I could put venous access and take blood in my sleep; I was very skilled at emergencies, at all of those things.
>
> But I moved out ten years ago doing mostly home births primarily because I was so distressed at what I was seeing happen to women, and I was becoming a part of it. I found I thought I'd walk into there as the expert, but I walked into there having to unlearn so many bad habits. I found that the first few home births that I was at I could not sit still.
>
> I was with really experienced home birth midwives who pulled out their knitting and knitted away, and I was used to running up and down delivery ward corridors being the efficient, competent midwife, and the efficient, competent midwife was the busy one. And suddenly I'm in a woman's home for seventeen hours listening to Enya and smelling

candles, and I was just beside myself, so I ended up having to take up crocheting (I'm not a good knitter) to stop myself, to take my adrenaline down, and to make me present.

It took me a couple of years to unlearn the rush of midwifery and learn that the art of just simply being there is one of the most powerful tools a midwife has.

Now I love it. I love the lights all dim, the music's playing, the dog's sitting by the fire, the children are playing in their pajamas, and I am home.

I also had to relearn the way I related, because I was used to obstetric beds. I was used to the bright lights. I was used to women not functioning physiologically. So I had to relearn women's progress signs as we weren't doing vaginal examinations regularly.

We were doing them if women wanted. I had to start learning the external signs a woman gives you, rather than always depending on how many centimeters she was. So for me, that expert midwife had a very hard lesson, that the most expert midwife was the one who sits and watches and learns from women.

Home birth is an amazing contrast to the hectic, frenetic pace most labor and delivery units operate under. The calm ambience at a home birth is a wonderful experience for the mother and baby.

While some women choose to have a home birth for reasons of comfort, other women specifically choose a home birth because of an aversion to hospitals. This aversion may be from a prior negative birth experience. It may also stem from an association with a medical hospitalization, either from their own illness or a close family member's illness. In this situation, they just can't imagine birthing their baby at the hospital because of all the negative associations and memories.

Another motive for a home birth is to avoid exposing yourself and your baby to hospital germs. This reasoning is especially valid in light of the COVID-19 outbreak. There is a real risk of picking up illnesses while in the hospital. The term for this is nosocomial infection[6], also known as Hospital Acquired Infection (HAI). These infections are introduced through patients and are circulated in the hospital by hospital staff rotating between patients and units. Having a baby at home means not having to worry about picking up a nosocomial infection from the maternity unit or newborn nursery[7].

Our own homes contain "friendly bacteria[8]," which are bacteria we are accustomed to and therefore do not cause us harm.

"Home births have much lower infection rates. We rarely have infections at home," points out Leah Marinelli[9], a home birth midwife.

Home birth midwives are diligent about following proper hygiene practices. Therefore, it is rare to pick up an infection during a home birth.

When deciding if a home birth is right for you, it is worthwhile to explore Jerome Groopman and Pamela Hartzbands' book *Your Medical Mind*[10], which categorizes people according to their approach to medical treatment. They contrast the following categories:

- Naturalist vs. Technologist
- Minimalist vs. Maximalist
- Doubter vs. Believer

Naturalists see the natural world as a safe and effective source of cures and remedies. Naturalists will utilize herbs and supplements to treat illnesses and will only turn to western medicine as a last resort.

Technologists believe the advancement of science and technology are key in combatting illness and disease. Technology is a gift that should be utilized to the greatest extent possible.

Minimalists believe the body is primed to heal itself and needs little help in the process. They don't take much notice of aches and pains and rarely see a doctor. They feel the less treatment they accept, the better.

Maximalists are people who extensively research their symptoms. They seek out all options to find relief from their maladies.

A doubter is someone who is skeptical of any medical treatment. They are concerned about the side effects of drugs and question their health care provider's recommendations.

A believer is someone who strongly favors medical intervention and treatments. They hold health care providers in great esteem, respecting their knowledge and expertise. Believers rely on medical professionals to do what they feel is best.

Which categories do you feel you fit into?

Think about it:

How do you approach your aches and pains? What's your first impulse when feeling sick? Do you reach out to your doctor immediately, or do you first reach for your naturopathic remedies?

As you approach the birth of your child, how will your natural inclination influence your decision?

For example, you might be a minimalist technologist where you don't want any medical interventions but still want to birth in a hospital so that the technology is there if needed.

You may be a maximalist technologist and want as many sensors and machines as possible. You may only feel comfortable in a major medical center with a high level NICU. Or you may be a minimalist naturalist and prefer letting nature takes its course in an unmedicalized, natural setting.

While your peace of mind is vital when choosing the right setting to birth your baby, it is important to be fully aware of all the possibilities and available options. For some, that peace of mind can be found in the hospital, and for others, that peace of mind can be found at home.

CHAPTER 2

How Does Your Body Birth a Baby?

Birthing your baby is a complex process that begins in your cervix. Your cervix[11] is the neck of your uterus. Early on in pregnancy, your cervix forms a mucus plug, sealing the uterus off from the vagina. It is like the cork plugging up the long neck of a wine bottle. The mucus plug works as a barrier to keep out bacteria[12] and viruses that may cause infection.

Toward the end of your pregnancy, your cervix will change. Imagine a glass bottle containing a large ship inside it, and you want to get that ship out. A few things have to take place to make it happen. Firstly, your cervix softens and ripens, thinning out in a process called effacement[13]. Before your cervix effaces, it is at 0% effacement and as it effaces, it progresses to 100% effacement.

At 0% effacement, your cervix feels similar to the tip of your nose. As it effaces, it becomes softer and thinner until it melts into your uterine wall, and you can't actually feel it anymore. The mucus plug or, in our example, the cork in the bottle, will release during effacement. Some women don't actually see it as it may break up and dissolve slowly.

Once effacement is complete, instead of a long neck to your wine bottle, you will have no neck.

Now, your bottle opening needs to widen. This occurs as your cervix dilates from 0 to 10 centimeters in a process called dilatation. The work of dilating your cervix is performed through uterine contractions. Some women have Braxton-Hicks contractions during pregnancy. Braxton-Hicks contractions are mildly uncomfortable but don't actually dilate your cervix. It is more like your uterus doing a workout to get itself in shape before a big marathon. These practice contractions are squeezing the uterus around the middle, which may be uncomfortable but are not painful. Contractions that dilate your cervix are concentrated at the fundus, which is the top of your uterus, as the contractions pull the uterus up forcing the bottom opening to widen. At the beginning, these contractions will feel like heavy menstrual cramps, and you may even feel them in your lower back. These early contractions may start out around 30 minutes apart and last 30 to 45 seconds. They will eventually pick up until they come every 3 to 5 minutes and last 60 to 90 seconds.

During labor, your body is releasing the hormone oxytocin, which stimulates the uterus to contract. The intensity and frequency of contractions mirror the rise of oxytocin in your blood stream, with contractions increasing in frequency and intensity as labor progresses. As labor progresses and oxytocin levels rise, many women report feeling their perception of time and space changing[14]. Their minds turn inward as they focus exclusively on the task of birthing their baby.

As your baby moves down, it passes through a sturdy ring of bones that encloses and protects your uterus and other lower abdominal organs. Your baby will pass specific markers, called stations. The stations measure from -3 to +3, depending on where the lowest part of the baby's head is relative to your pelvis. Your baby starts out at -3 station, which is when your baby has not yet moved into your pelvis. Each marker is a centimeter apart from there, so your baby will move from -3 to -2 to -1 to 0 station. Zero station is when your baby's head reaches the middle of your pelvis, a position also known as "engaged." Your baby's head becomes engaged in the pelvis during "lightening," which is when you feel your baby dropping low in your abdomen. This transpires at some point within the last two weeks of pregnancy, although with moms who have previously given birth, their baby may not drop until labor begins. When that happens, your baby bump will appear lower down than it did before the baby "dropped." As labor progresses and contractions intensify, your baby will move down from +1 to +2. Once your baby is at +3 station, your baby's head will be "crowning," which is when the baby's head emerges from the mother's vagina.

There are three stages to labor:
- Stage 1 is when the cervix dilates from 0 to 10 centimeters.
- Stage 2 is the birth of your baby.
- Stage 3 is the delivery of placenta.

Stage 1: Cervical Dilatation
The first stage is by far the longest, and it is broken down into three phases.

Phase 1- Early Labor

The first phase occurs as the cervix dilates from 0 to 4 centimeters. Contractions may be coming every 5 to 20 minutes and last 30 to 60 seconds. This phase may last from 12 hours up to several days. You will feel some discomfort but will still be able to walk around, talk, and carry on with your regular activities in between contractions.

Phase 2- Active Labor

The second phase is when the cervix dilates from 5 to 715 centimeters. Contractions start becoming more intense and will last between 45 to 60 seconds. Once you hit 616 centimeters, contractions will come consistently every 2 to 5 minutes. Phase 2 may last 6 hours or more, but it marks the transition from latent labor to active labor, when a woman begins to realize "this is it."

If your water hasn't broken yet, it will usually break during this phase. Some mothers may lose their appetite and feel nauseous. You may turn inward and not speak much, and at this point, you may want to begin using the labor coping techniques that you prepared.

Phase 3- Transition

The third phase is called transition, and it is the final phase of labor. Contractions may last 60 to 90 seconds and are very powerful. They come every 2 to 3 minutes and you may feel a lot of pressure on your lower back from the baby's head moving down. Some women get very hot, sweat profusely, and experience uncontrollable shaking; some women may even vomit. This is usually the point when a woman feels like she can't go on any longer. This is usually a clue that your baby will be here very soon. This phase can last from several minutes up to 2 hours.

Stage 2: Birth

Stage 2 is the birth of your baby. It is also known as the "pushing phase." Most women are relieved when they can begin bearing down and actively moving their baby out. Some moms may have a resting phase[17] that begins when they reach 10 centimeters dilation. This is where contractions cease completely for about a half hour to an hour. It is the body's way of regaining its energy before pushing the baby out.

Rachel's Story

Rachel labored for several hours as her contractions intensified. As her belly tightened and then released, Rachel replayed her birth mantras through her mind:

"My body opens wide, my baby descends."

"With each breath I come closer to meeting my baby."

"I've got this."

"This will not last forever."

Like a song set to repeat, the contractions kept coming.

And then nothing.

Rachel closed her eyes, grateful for the reprieve. Her birth companions, along with her baby, waited silently in anticipation. For 20 minutes all was still, and then Rachel opened her eyes and called out, "Baby's coming."

The midwife, gloved and ready, talked soothingly as Rachel pushed with the next contraction.

When Rachel's friend asked her in amazement what it felt like to push out her baby without having an epidural, Rachel responded, "It felt like a giant impacted stool." Rachel and her friend shared a laugh, but Rachel remembered how her body responded to the sensations she felt as she maneuvered onto her knees, crouching on a thick fleece blanket covering her floor. Rachel hugged a pillow with her forearms and bore down with the contraction. The force of her

contractions, coupled with concentrated pushing, propelled her baby neatly into
her midwife's waiting hands.

Women who are unmedicated during labor will feel the baby
moving down and the subsequent urge to push.

Once your baby is born, your provider will immediately assess
your baby's health using a grading system called an Apgar score[18].

APGAR stands for:
Activity
Pulse
Grimace
Appearance
Respiration

Every baby gets a score of 0, 1, or 2 per category.

Activity is graded 2 for active movement and 1 for some
movement.

Pulse is graded 2 for heart rate above 100 and 1 for heart rate
below 100.

Grimace is graded 2 for sneezing, coughing, or pulling away
when stimulated and 1 for grimace or feeble cry when stimulated.

Appearance is graded 2 for no blue coloration and 1 for blue
extremities. Normally, babies' extremities are slightly bluish, so a
score of 1 in the category of Appearance is normal.

Respiration is graded 2 for strong cry and 1 for weak, slow, or
irregular breathing.

The Apgar scoring system is an easy way to communicate
between providers regarding the well-being of the baby at birth.
Each baby is graded once at birth and then again five minutes later.
An Apgar score of 9 or 10 is good.

It's important to keep in mind, though, that Apgar scores do not predict the future health of the baby. They are solely for an initial assessment of the baby and its adjustment to life outside the womb. Many babies have poor Apgar scores at birth but then go on to develop normally.

Stage 3: Delivering the Placenta

After your baby is born, uterine contractions help the placenta separate from the uterine wall and pass through the vagina.

The placenta[19] is a miraculous organ that attaches to the uterine wall and serves as a conduit between mom and baby. It provides nourishment to the baby through the umbilical cord, which is a thick cord connecting baby to the mother. The umbilical cord contains one vein carrying oxygen and nutrient rich blood to the baby from the placenta, and two arteries carrying waste from baby to the placenta to be eliminated through the mother's circulation. With the birth of the baby the placenta's job is done. It comes out soft and squishy, usually within thirty minutes of the baby's birth.

Sarah's Story

After Sarah birthed her baby, she cradled her on her belly as her midwife clamped and cut the cord. As her baby squirmed around, Sarah felt some strong period cramps and then felt something soft slide between her legs. Her midwife caught her placenta in a basin and looked at it carefully to make sure all parts of the placenta were there.

One side of the placenta was white, shiny, and smooth, which was the side facing the baby in utero. The other side was made up of 20 to 25 small cups called cotyledons. These cotyledons were attached to the uterine wall. Her midwife carefully inspected the placenta to make sure that no pieces were left inside.

Sarah felt some gushes of blood. Her midwife checked the bleeding and determined it was a normal amount and her uterus was firm. Sarah continued to feel contractions and asked for ibuprofen. Sarah's midwife gave her some and told her she will continue to feel heavy period cramps over the next few days as her uterus contracts down to size. Contractions would intensify during breastfeeding, as breastfeeding releases the hormone oxytocin which causes uterine contractions. Contractions minimize postpartum bleeding. Sarah took ibuprofen a half hour before breastfeeding for the first few days to ease the cramps. As the days went by, the contractions diminished in intensity until she didn't feel them anymore. Bleeding from the site where the placenta was attached to the uterus, also called lochia, continues intermittently for up to six weeks after birth.

CHAPTER 3

The Truth About Doctors, Hospitals, and Medical Interventions

S hannon's Story
Shannon excitedly planned a home birth for her second child's birth. Her first child had been born via c-section, and she was hoping to avoid a repeat. She anticipated a VBAC (pronounced v-back), which is an abbreviation for "vaginal birth after cesarean." VBAC home births are often successful, but a woman who wants one needs to be carefully screened by her midwife to ensure it is safe. The circumstances surrounding the initial c-section, as well as the course of the postpartum recovery, may preclude a home birth. Shannon's midwife agreed to take her on as a home birth client, and Shannon took a hypnobirthing class to prepare.

Shannon went into labor and her midwife came over as her contractions picked up. Another midwife joined soon after, and Shannon noticed her midwives granted her far more autonomy at her home birth than she had previously experienced at the hospital.

At Shannon's first birth, doctors restricted her movement and confined her to her hospital bed. Unable to manage her contractions while lying on her back, she requested an epidural anesthesia. Shannon received an IV, and the anesthesiologist inserted the epidural catheter. The medication flowed in, providing instant relief from the intense contractions. However, her doctor started her on a Pitocin drip to keep the contractions going and to move her labor along. From there, her baby developed distress, and Shannon found herself in the operating room having a c-section.

Now experiencing her second birth, Shannon focused her mind on riding the waves of contractions. Her midwife encouraged her to follow her instincts. There were no constraints; she was free to move around at will. Knowing everyone present in her home while she labored soothed her and freed her mind to focus on the work of labor.

Shannon moved through the phases of labor and birthed her baby with ease while supported and in control. Shannon's birth experience transformed her and soothed that part of herself that thought her incapable of birthing her own child naturally. She knew she could do it, and she did.

Shannon's story contrasts two birth settings, as well as highlights the difference between doctor's care and midwifery care. Home birth and hospital birth are vastly different from one another.

"Women who have babies at a hospital and then have a home birth will tell me it's like two completely different experiences," comments Mrs. Yetty Engel, CM[20], a home birth midwife in New York.

The major difference between these two settings is the heavy influence of doctors on a hospital birth. Doctors guide hospital policy and protocol, and they favor strict monitoring and routine intervention during labor.

Midwives, on the other hand, monitor as necessary but are less inclined to intervene unless medically indicated. In a hospital setting, their authority remains limited. In Israel, where midwives are the primary caregivers for low-risk births in the hospital, doctors directly influence hospital culture. Midwife Mindy Levy[21] describes:

> They are two completely different professions. The approach is completely different. It's a problem because midwives basically manage all the low-risk births, and the doctors manage all the high-risk births. But in a doctor's mind, every low-risk birth is a potential high-risk birth.
>
> Instead of the doctor sitting outside and saying, "I trust you. I'm sure everything is going to be fine. If you need me, call me," they're lurking all the time. They're sticking their noses in, and poking, and telling the midwives what to do. They're telling them to cut an episiotomy, to break the water, and to do all kinds of things that have nothing to do with them.

The field of obstetrics and gynecology is a relatively new field, only about 200 years old. According to the book *Birth: The Surprising History of How We Are Born*[22], by Tina Cassidy, the word "obstetrician" was coined by an English doctor in 1828. The Latin root is shared with the word "obstruct," which means "to stand before," or "in the way." The first obstetricians were male barbers who used forceps to deliver babies. These obstetricians educated other men on utilizing instruments to birth babies, and thus, the profession of obstetrics was born. From the earliest initiation of male-led obstetrics, the obstetrician was encouraged to actively deliver the baby, as opposed to watchfully waiting as the birth process unfolds.

In the early 1900s, obstetrics as a subspecialty of medicine was looked down upon by other doctors in the medical profession. At the time, most births were attended by midwives, and obstetrics was viewed as a profession which didn't require any real skill or education. Birthing a baby was a normal, natural occurrence so why would a doctor who possessed great talent and knowledge of medicine need to be present? It was considered inauthentic medicine.

Dr. DeLee[23], an American obstetrician in the early 1900s, made it his life's work to elevate the obstetric profession, and he became known as the father of modern obstetrics. Dr. DeLee built up the profession, taking a non-medical life event, and medicalizing it. He felt that the reason obstetrics was looked down upon was because it was considered "normal," which, therefore, meant anyone could deliver a baby. He set out to prove that only doctors had the specialized skill and knowledge to safely deliver a baby. He labeled midwives "incompetent" and cautioned women that they could only birth their babies safely under a physician's care.

He advocated prophylactically removing the baby from the birth canal before any indication of help was needed. He believed it was in the best interest of the mother to intervene routinely as soon as full cervical dilation was achieved. He popularized episiotomies, where a cut is made to the vagina in order to widen the opening. The doctor then used forceps to draw the baby out of the birth canal. He also instituted "twilight sleep," by giving moms a cocktail of drugs so that they wouldn't remember any of it.

Just like medicine focuses on preventing illness and disease, Dr. DeLee hoped to bring that approach to childbirth. This well-meaning philosophy is at the heart of obstetrics today. Instead of responding to problems as they arise, doctors routinely intervene throughout labor.

One of the greatest impacts Dr. DeLee has had on childbirth in the United States is the removal of care of childbearing women from midwives to obstetricians.

Despite beginning the tradition of heavily medicalized births, Dr. DeLee made an important contribution when he succeeded in having obstetrics accepted into mainstream medicine. Obstetricians today are a blessing and they save lives every day. If a risk factor presents itself during pregnancy or birth, or for a woman with a preexisting medical condition, an obstetrician can provide the safe care they need to birth their baby.

The obstetric profession also produced doctors like Dr. Dick-Read, Dr. Lamaze, and Dr. Bradley, who reintroduced the idea that woman can manage birth naturally and without medication.

Dr. Dick-Read published a book in 1942 called *Childbirth Without Fear*[24], where he brought back the idea of natural birth. He wrote, "It is as great a crime to leave a woman alone in her agony and deny her relief from her suffering, as it is to insist upon dulling the consciousness of a natural mother who desires above all things to be aware of the final reward of her efforts, whose ambition is to be present, in full possession of her senses, when the infant she already adores greets her with its first loud cry and the soft touch of its restless body upon her limbs." Dr. Dick-Read spoke out against forcibly anesthetizing women during labor, which was commonly practiced at the time.

Dr. Lamaze[25], a French obstetrician on whose teachings Lamaze classes are based, taught in the 1950s that it is possible to birth a baby and manage contractions without drugs. He advocated using a specific breathing technique that induces relaxation, as well as distracts from painful contractions. Dr. Lamaze brought back the idea that women can birth their babies without requiring medication, and with the ability to be mentally present in the moment of their child's birth.

In 1962 Dr. Bradley[26] published "Fathers' Presence in Delivery Rooms," which was considered radical at the time. He advocated having husbands at their wife's side during labor and birth, coaching and supporting them through natural childbirth. It was a novel idea for the time, even scandalous, as until that time fathers were never permitted in the delivery room while a woman birthed her baby. It was termed *"The Bradley Method"*, and the fact that fathers are welcomed and expected to stay and support their wives throughout labor and birth is attributed to Dr. Bradley.

While some obstetricians have helped bring back the concept of natural birth, mainstream obstetrics continues to employ protocols that have not been proven to produce good birth outcomes. They rely on tradition and routines instead of evidence-based medicine. Evidence-based medicine is a common-sense method of practicing medicine where only treatment and interventions that are proven successful are performed. This method is standardized in general medicine, and there is a movement to bring evidence-based medicine into the obstetrics profession as well.

For example, women who birth upright and change positions at will have a shorter labor and a reduced risk for perineal tears than women who labor on their backs.

A woman laboring on her back cannot utilize the force of gravity to bring her baby down. Being in the upright position will allow gravity to aid the baby's descent through the birth canal, giving the baby direction as it moves into the optimal position for birth. Gravity also keeps the pressure of the baby's head on the cervix, softening and dilating it.

For these reasons, labor moves slower when a woman is lying on her back. A Cochrane review[27] published in 2014 found that, on average, a woman's labor was prolonged by an hour when she labored on her back.

When labor is not moving forward efficiently, doctors perform c-sections for "failure to progress." In 2014, the percentage of c-sections caused by failure to progress was 35%[28]. The c-section rate in the United States today is over 30%, so about 10% of women who are having a baby end up with a c-section due to failure to progress.

In 2015, a CNN report[29] showed that maternal mortality rates in the United States doubled between 1990 and 2008, the same time period when the c-section rate[30] increased from 20% to 32%.

If the c-section rate in the United States is 32%,[31] this means that 1 in every 3 births is a c-section. The World Health Organization (WHO)[32] recommends c-section rates should ideally be between 10 to 15%, which means the United States has a c-section rate that is double the recommended rate. Some countries like Brazil, Egypt, Dominican Republic, and Turkey have a c-section rate that is over 50%.[33]

Unfortunately, a country's high c-section rate indicates that many c-sections are performed unnecessarily. The American College of Obstetricians and Gynecologists (ACOG) [34] put out a statement in March 2014 indicating that the rise of c-sections in the United States from 1996 to 2011 with no reduction in maternal or fetal mortality raised concern that c-sections are overdone. It was recommended that obstetricians revise their justification for c-sections. Moreover, Dr. Neel Shah, Assistant Professor of Obstetrics, Gynecology and Reproductive Biology, at the Harvard Medical School, wrote the following lines in an article published on June 3, 2015 in *The Conversation:*[35]

Cesareans are designed to be a lifesaving surgery, but they are now so routine that c-sections have become the most common major surgery performed on human beings. It hasn't been until recently that we started to fully consider the downside of Caesarean deliveries.

For starters, caring for a newborn while dealing with a 12-centimeter skin incision in your own abdomen is the pits, especially when compared to caring for a newborn without having a 12-centimeter skin incision.

Though common, let's not forget that c-sections are a major abdominal surgery that can lead to threefold higher rates of serious complications for mothers compared to vaginal delivery (2.7 percent vs 0.9 percent). These complications can include severe infection, organ injury and hemorrhage. I should also point out that the first c-section a woman has is an easy surgery- I can train an intern to do one safely in just a few weeks. But most women have more than one child, and most women who have a c-section the first time will have a c-section the next time. Obstetricians are among a small group of surgeons who regularly operate on the same part of the same patient over and over again, dissecting thicker layers of old scar tissue with each surgery. By the second, third, or fourth c-section on the same patient, the anatomy becomes distorted and the surgery becomes increasingly technical. I recently did a cesarean where the woman's abdominal muscles, bladder and uterus were fused together like a melted box of crayons.

In the most dreaded cases, a woman's placenta (a large bag of blood vessels that nourishes the fetus) can get stuck in this mess of tissue and fail to detach normally. In these cases, pints of blood may be lost within minutes, and the only way to stop the bleeding is often to do a hysterectomy.

C-sections should only be done if absolutely necessary because of the risks to mother and baby. Damage to internal organs can occur by way of surgical accidents, and bladders have been nicked on occasion. About 1%[36] of babies born via c-section suffer injuries from the surgeon's knife. For moms, additional risks[37] that come along with c-sections include internal bleeding, blood clots, hemorrhage, and infection.

Mothers who undergo c-sections[38] take longer to recover than mothers who have had vaginal births. Pain at the surgical site is typical and may take from weeks to months to resolve. In addition, women who have had a c-section are at risk for placental abnormalities during future pregnancies, namely placenta accreta[39] where the placenta grows too deeply into the uterine wall and does not detach normally at birth. Placenta accreta can cause significant hemorrhaging at birth and is not always picked up by ultrasound prior to birth. The most important risk factor for this condition is a prior c-section. Placenta accreta[40] used to occur in 1 in 30,000 births in the 1950s,[41] but it is now 1 in 500 births[42]. The incidence of placenta accreta has gone up with the rising c-section rate.

What is your chance of having a c-section? It really depends on your doctor and the hospital you are giving birth in. Besides your provider's c-section rate, every hospital has its own c-section rate. Both factors will influence your odds of having one. A 2017 Consumers Report[43] analysis of more than 1300 hospitals in the United States showed a wide range of c-section rates. Rates varied from 7% to 51%, with large differences found even within the same zip code.

Every hospital obstetric unit has protocols that doctors must follow in order to continue practicing there. Not all of the protocols are in the best interests of mother and baby, but are put in place in order to prevent lawsuits. Some of those protocols interfere with the progress of labor and can cause unnecessary c-sections.

In 2015, the *British Medical Journal*[44] released a study where data from acute care hospitals in Florida was reviewed between the years 2000 and 2009. They looked to see if doctors who drive up hospital costs by ordering many tests were associated with a lower incidence of malpractice claims. Seven specialties were covered, including obstetrics.

Across the specialties, they found that doctors who ordered more tests and interventions had fewer malpractice claims. Specifically in obstetrics, they found that the higher a doctor's c-section rate, the lower the incidence of lawsuits. The fact of the matter is, very few lawsuits are brought against a doctor performing an unnecessary c-section. Unfortunately, a high c-section rate indicates unnecessary c-sections are being done.

Many obstetricians approach childbirth hyperaware of the risk for a lawsuit that hangs over every birth. Of course you want them to practice safe medicine, but logically, safe practices are practices that are proven with evidence. For example, continuous EFM (Electronic Fetal Monitor) is required by some doctors and hospitals as a means of defensive medicine. An EFM consists of an electronic fetal monitor with 2 belts, each of which has a monitor attached. One monitor measures the intensity and duration of uterine contractions. The other monitor records the fetal heart rate.

In a court of law[45], it is standard of care to have an EFM tracing. This means that if a doctor is sued after a baby is born with cerebral palsy, they may lose the case if there is no EFM tracing.

This may occur even if it is a low-risk pregnancy where there is no indication for wearing an EFM during labor. Unfortunately, because of this reality, there are many women who are denied the right to move around and to assume a position that is more conducive for a natural safer birth during labor. This is the conundrum doctors face. Even if the doctor doesn't believe an intervention is absolutely necessary, and would like to give their patient the choice to have an EFM or not, they feel the pressure to cover themselves. Many obstetricians would like to implement evidence-based practices, but find themselves walking a fine line in order not to suffer retribution by colleagues and the hospitals they practice in. They may tell you, privately, that they support unmedicated childbirth, but will they allow you to labor in a way that will promote it?

I know someone who was seeing an obstetrician for a planned hospital birth who related, "I told the doctor I didn't want an IV during labor, and he answered: 'Sorry, I'm not going to war with the entire nursing staff for one patient.'"

I have personally witnessed nurses remind midwives of hospital protocol, and then stay in the room to make sure they are following it. It is unfortunate that there is a disparity between what evidence shows is best practice and hospital protocol.

EFM tracings indicating signs of fetal distress is a common reason to do a c-section, but it is not the most common. The most common reason to do a c-section in the United States is because labor "is taking too long[46]." There are different reasons why labor may be prolonged, some very valid. For example, a woman may have cephalopelvic disproportion (CPD), where her pelvis is too narrow for a typically sized baby, or the baby is too big to fit through a normal sized pelvis. In this situation, the only way to deliver the baby is via c-section. This accounts for 0.3%[47] of women.

In a similar situation, a c-section is necessary when the baby descends at an awkward angle and gets stuck behind a bony prominence of its mother's pelvis. No matter how much time they give the baby, there is no progress. In this scenario, the mother would require a c-section to deliver her baby.

Often though, women are simply not given enough time to labor. This is especially true of women giving birth for the first time; first-time moms tend to have longer labors than women who've previously given birth.

The Friedman Curve[48] was the first graph showing the variability in the progression of normal labor. In 1955, Dr. Friedman, an American obstetrician, graphed the length of women's labor on a bell chart. He then used that chart to come up with a set of averages for the length of the different stages of labor. He published his findings in order to identify when women were having a longer-than-average labor.

Over time, the terms "failure to progress" and "labor dystocia[49]," were given to describe labor that fell on the lower end of the bell curve. In the last few decades, these terms came to be considered enough of a reason to perform a c-section.

This graph sets a norm that the first stage of labor should follow, namely that cervical dilatation should progress 1 centimeter per hour. This "rule" has since been disproven by a number of studies that show mothers and babies both do well, even if their labor runs a little longer. There has also been a movement to consider active labor beginning at 6 centimeters, as that is usually when dilation becomes more consistent. This way, interventions can be held off for a little longer, which gives the mother the opportunity to progress at her own pace.

If you're planning a hospital birth, it is best to stay home[50] for as long as possible when you're in labor. Women labor better and progress more rapidly when they are in a familiar environment. This way, your labor will be well underway by the time you get to the hospital. Of course, please be in touch with your health care provider during labor to determine the best time to go to the hospital.

CHAPTER 4
What are Common Hospital Protocols?

Kate's Story
Kate arrives at the hospital after an uncomfortable car ride with regular contractions. She breathes through her contractions while answering questions at the hospital registration desk (even though she had preregistered). Finally, she's admitted. The nurse brings Kate into a room and has her lie down on a bed while she takes her vital signs. She attaches an electronic fetal monitor to Kate's belly to monitor her contractions and the baby's heart rate. Kate notices how much more intense the contractions are when she lies down. She breathes through them as she was taught. It helps for a little while, but then Kate's contractions become really uncomfortable and the breathing techniques aren't helping anymore. She is unable to do anything to relieve the pain as she is literally strapped to the bed.

Finally, Kate's doctor shows up, and after checking her, notes she is 4 centimeters dilated. He lets her know she is in active labor and may not eat or drink. He would like to give her IV fluids so that she does not get dehydrated. He also recommends getting an epidural for her comfort. Kate hadn't planned on getting an epidural, but with her pain escalating and her doctor wanting her to remain on a continuous fetal monitor, she doesn't think she'll be able to manage otherwise. Her husband, John, is feeling really bad for her and is unsure how to help; he encourages her to get the epidural.

Kate figures if the doctor recommends it, then it must be okay. Kate's nurse inserts the IV into her arm. The anesthesiologist comes by soon after and successfully inserts the epidural. Within moments, Kate feels relief and is happy to rest. Kate's doctor adds Pitocin to her IV as the contractions had slowed due to the epidural's effects. Once the Pitocin is added, Kate notices the contractions on the graph are peaking higher, lasting longer, and coming closer together. After a little while the nurse, who has been watching the electronic fetal monitor, walks out to let Kate's doctor know the baby is having decels, which are temporary drops in the baby's heart rate that may be a signal of the baby's distress.

Kate's doctor keeps an eye on the graph as he notes the baby's developing distress. He begins talking to Kate and John about performing a c-section, due to the baby's condition.

This scenario happens regularly in hospitals all around the country. It is called "the cascade of interventions[51]," which is a phrase describing how one intervention leads to another intervention that leads to another, which then leads to a c-section.

Interventions[52] that may begin this cascade include those performed at Kate's birth, such as having an IV, having a continuous electronic fetal monitor, restricting food and drink, and receiving Pitocin through an IV.

In a February 2018 release[53], the World Health Organization stated, "The prevailing model of intrapartum care in many parts of the world, which enables the health care provider to control the birthing process, may expose apparently healthy pregnant women to unnecessary medical interventions that interfere with the physiological process of childbirth."

Even minor medical interventions, like restricting movement during labor, disrupts the natural progression[54] of labor and birth.

One of the first interventions a woman will encounter when she enters the hospital is an electronic fetal monitor (EFM). EFM is favored in almost every hospital in the United States. Evidence Based Birth's[55] signature article on EFM discusses its origins and use. It was first introduced in the 1970s with claims it would reduce the incidence of cerebral palsy. It was thought that cerebral palsy was caused by reduced blood flow to the baby during labor, leading to oxygen deprivation[56] in the baby's brain. This theory has since been disproven as cerebral palsy rates[57] have remained the same[58] over the last few decades since EFM was introduced and adopted as the standard of care.

In February 2019, the American College of Obstetricians and Gynecologists (ACOG) stated in their Committee Opinion Number 766[59]: "Continuous EFM was introduced to reduce the incidence of perinatal death and cerebral palsy and as an alternative to the practice of intermittent auscultation. However, the widespread use of continuous EFM has not been shown to significantly affect such outcomes as perinatal death and cerebral palsy when used for women with low-risk pregnancies."

The United Kingdom's National Institute for Health and Care Excellence (NICE) [60] does not recommend cardiotocography (CTG), the term for EFM in England, for normally developing, low-risk labors. This is because of the increased risk for c-sections that is associated with EFM use. The question is, why?

There are several reasons.

For one, when an EFM is placed for continuous monitoring, the mother is now confined to bed and limited in how she can manage her contractions. Lying on your back is arguably the most uncomfortable and inefficient position to labor in. Women are much more likely to turn to an epidural if they have an EFM, and epidurals are associated with a higher rate[61] of c-sections.

Second, the vena cava is a large vein that brings nutrient rich blood to the uterus. When a woman is lying down on her back, the weight of the uterus may compress[62] the vein, which then reduces blood flow to the placenta and baby. The reduction in blood flow to the baby may result in an EFM tracing indicating fetal distress, and subsequently necessitate a c-section.

Lastly, EFM tracing may be unreliable[63], with the ability to read it accurately dependent on the skill of the doctor. It is entirely possible for a doctor to misinterpret a tracing as fetal distress and perform a c-section when, in fact, the baby was doing okay.

A September 2014 study by doctors from Johns Hopkins University in the *Journal of Obstetrics & Gynecology*[64], shows that EFM tracing was not a good predictor of fetal outcomes in the hour prior to delivery. Dr. Ernest Graham[65], one of the researchers of the study, said, "Brain injuries caused by oxygen deprivation in newborns are rare, and our study shows that in most cases, irregularities detected by an electronic heart rate monitor are false alarms."

In 2017, researchers in Norway published a study[66] on the changes ultrasound and EFM have had on infant mortality. They used data provided by the Medical Birth Registry of Norway for approximately 1.2 million births between the years 1967 and 1995. While they found a nearly 20% reduction in infant mortality with the use of ultrasound, they found no reduction in infant mortality using EFM technology.

Can EFM be helpful?

EFM tracks the baby's heart rate, and can detect the rare trauma that may occur in utero that causes the baby's heart rate to dramatically drop, such as placental abruption or uterine rupture.

In June 2011, the *American Journal of Gynecology*[67] published "Electronic Fetal Heart Rate Monitoring and its Relationship to Neonatal and Infant Mortality in the United States." The researchers used the 2004 US birth/infant death set assembled by the National Center for Health Statistics. They found that for full term births, 4,078 women would need to be kept on continuous EFM during labor in order to prevent one death. The study acknowledges the increased incidence of c-sections associated with EFM.

Are there any alternatives to EFM?

An alternative method to EFM is intermittent auscultation[68], where the provider listens to the baby's heart rate periodically during labor. The most common instrument used is a Doppler, or a fetoscope, which is a machine similar to an ultrasound, but it is handheld and only measures the baby's heartbeat. Another instrument is a Pinard, which is a horn-shaped instrument constructed from wood.

Intermittent auscultation gives you the ability to move freely in labor, while at the same time allowing the midwife or doctor to monitor the baby. It solves the problem of restricting movement. If so, are there any benefits to using continuous EFM over intermittent auscultation during labor?

I did find one benefit in a Cochrane Review[69] published in the UK in 2017. The review surveyed 13 trials involving 37,000 women. It showed no difference in neonatal mortality or cerebral palsy rates, whether women were on continuous EFM or intermittent auscultation. It did show, however, that moms who were on continuous EFM had a 50% reduction in neonatal seizures compared to moms who had intermittent auscultation.

Incidence of seizures in full term newborns is between 1.8 and 5 per 1000 births[70]. The incidence varies depending on the circumstances of the baby's birth. For example, if a baby is born premature, they have a greater risk of developing newborn seizures. Newborn seizures may cause no harm to the infant or they may have long term neuropsychological effects[71], but there has not been enough follow-up research done to confirm this.

The World Health Organization published a statement[72] on February 15, 2018 that continuous EFM is not recommended for healthy women with normally developing labor. Another statement[73] released on February 17, 2018 stated: "Intermittent auscultation of the fetal heart rate with either a Doppler ultrasound device or a Pinard fetal stethoscope is recommended for healthy pregnant women in labour."

Eating & Drinking

Most hospitals have an NPO policy for women in labor. NPO is a Latin abbreviation for "nothing by mouth." Basically, women are not allowed to eat or drink while they are in labor. This was instituted in 1946 by Dr Curtis Mendelson[74] during a time when women would be anesthetized into a "twilight sleep" when having their baby. When women were sedated in this manner, they found that if there was food or drink in their stomach, they were at risk of aspirating. Aspiration is when food or drink is inhaled into the lungs, causing breathing difficulties. This occurrence was termed Mendelson's Syndrome[75].

Nowadays, women are not sedated into a "twilight sleep." Doctors reason that restricting women from eating or drinking while in labor is important in case of an emergency c-section taking place under general anesthesia. The occurrence of a woman requiring an emergency c-section under general anesthesia and then aspirating during the birth is extremely rare, with one study[76] finding the risk to be 7 in 10 million births.

Many advocates for allowing women to eat and drink while in labor cite that not eating and drinking during labor causes hunger, thirst, exhaustion, low energy, and fatigue. In 2015, the American Society of Anesthesiologists released a paper[77] on this topic. The authors state that after researching the occurrence of aspiration during labor, they felt it necessary to completely revise their recommendation on eating and drinking during labor, as the occurrence of aspiration in labor is so rare. The authors recommend a light meal for healthy, low-risk women while they are in labor, comparing women in labor to marathon runners. The uterus uses large amounts of energy as it contracts, and adequate food and drink are needed to keep mom hydrated and energized.

Drinking throughout labor is also associated with a shorter labor[78]. An article published in the *American Journal of Obstetrics & Gynecology* in 2016[79] found no benefits to restricting eating and drinking during labor. The authors concluded the article by advocating for low-risk women to eat and drink freely while in labor. Although most women in labor will not feel like eating a heavy meal during labor, light snacks like yogurt, nuts, and fruit will give women the protein and complex carbohydrates they need for energy.

IVs

Inserting an IV is routine in many hospitals, and is performed when a woman is admitted to the labor and delivery unit. The IV provides hydration as women are typically restricted from eating and drinking during labor. In addition, in case an emergency c-section is needed, the IV is already in place. In many hospitals epidural anesthesia is so common that it's routine to receive an IV on admission in preparation for the epidural.

What are the downsides to receiving an IV?

Firstly, it's uncomfortable.

Second, once a mother is receiving IV fluids, her movement is restricted. She can't shower with it, and she does have to be aware of it when she moves around as it can get tangled or pulled if she's not careful.

In addition, the amount of IV fluid she receives can be too much, and the kidneys cannot flush out the excess fluid right away. This leads to fluid retention, where fluid ends up pooling under the skin in a condition known as edema. You can see the swelling in the ankles, abdomen, hands, fingers, and other areas. The baby may have difficulty latching on if the breasts are swollen due to the extra fluid. When a baby cannot latch onto the breast properly, the breasts will not be adequately stimulated, leading to a poor milk supply. It can actually take several weeks for the swelling to subside, as the body already has the extra fluid from the pregnancy to flush out.

Besides the mom retaining excess fluids, the American Academy of Pediatrics (AAP)[80] found that newborns whose mothers received IV fluid during labor had excessive weight loss after birth, as they shed the extra fluid they absorbed from their mothers during labor. This may raise concern on the pediatrician's side if the baby seems to be losing too much weight right after birth.

Breaking the Water

Breaking the water, also called artificial rupture of membranes (AROM), seems like a really easy way to jumpstart labor and kick things off. The upside is it usually does get things moving. This is because there are prostaglandins in the amniotic fluid which strengthen uterine contractions. As the amniotic fluid leaks out, contractions will become more intense. At the same time, the baby will lose the water cushion and will subsequently feel the contractions more intensely.

How do they break the water?

The health care provider takes an amnihook, which looks something like a crochet hook, and slides it through the vagina and tears the membranes holding the water and baby.

The problem with AROM is that once a woman's water breaks, the clock starts ticking. The more time passes after the water breaks, the greater the risk for infection. Infection occurs when bacteria migrates up the vagina into the uterus, causing chorioamnionitis[81]. This is an infection of the membranes surrounding the baby and the amniotic fluid. Many doctors will perform a c-section if the baby isn't born within 24 hours, to avoid the increased risk of infection.

AROM also carries a slight risk for cord prolapse[82], which is where the umbilical cord slips down into the vagina. Cord prolapse is a medical emergency as the cord can kink and cut off blood supply to the baby. In this situation, an emergency c-section is necessary. There is a 0.2% chance[83] of cord prolapse if AROM occurs, with the risk increasing the earlier in labor the provider breaks the water. AROM should only be done if the baby's head is engaged in the pelvis. This way, the opening of the uterus is blocked by the baby's head, with little room for the cord to slip through.

Epidurals

Epidurals are the most effective form of pain management for women in childbirth. An epidural is started by inserting a needle containing a small plastic catheter threaded behind it into the epidural space in a woman's back. It is a very precise procedure, and the woman has to remain still for about 5 minutes while the anesthesiologist inserts it and gets it into place. The needle is then removed and the catheter remains. Medication flows through the catheter and blocks pain signals from reaching the brain.

A CSE is a combined spinal epidural. This is the most popular method of administering an epidural. A smaller spinal needle is placed within the epidural needle, and medication is pushed through into the spinal space before it reaches the epidural space. The spinal gives moms immediate relief, and the epidural catheter is then set up and starts working within 15 minutes.

Some women go into labor planning on having an epidural, while for some women, it is something they choose after they have been in labor for a while.

Amanda's Story

Amanda had labored for 24 hours at home. She was completely wiped out, going on barely any sleep. Her midwife checked her and found she was only dilated 4 centimeters. Feeling really dispirited, Amanda cried that she couldn't go on anymore. Amanda's midwife reviewed her options with her, including going into the hospital for an epidural. Amanda and her husband discussed the pros and cons and ultimately decided she really needed that break. Once Amanda was admitted and received an epidural, her midwife urged her to rest, shutting the lights on her way out. Amanda and her husband closed their eyes and slept uninterrupted for 2 hours. They were thrilled when they woke up and found she was almost fully dilated.

For women in prolonged labor, like Amanda, an epidural may make sense. For someone completely exhausted and wrung out, a chance to rest and recoup their energy may outweigh the risks.

An epidural can give mom the chance to relax, which allows her cervix to dilate. Resting will also give mom renewed energy for the pushing phase.

There are several downsides to an epidural. One downside is that there are no guarantees it'll work. About 1%[84] of women who receive an epidural do not have sufficient pain relief and still feel the contractions.

There are additional side effects to epidurals:

Epidural Fever

About 23% of women who have an epidural develop fever during labor, compared to about 7% of women who develop fever during labor without an epidural. It is unknown why women with epidurals develop fever.

A February 2012 study[85] showed lower Apgar scores for babies whose mothers developed fever during labor. These babies were more likely to have low tone, need assistance breathing, and develop early onset seizures. Some hospital protocols require a newborn whose mothers had fever during labor to be observed in the NICU for a period of time after the birth, even if they are doing well. Some providers will treat a fever with antibiotics, both for the mother and for the baby, just in case the fever is related to an infection.

Low Blood Pressure

About 14%[86] of women who have an epidural also suffer a drop in their blood pressure. This can make them feel faint and light-headed. When a woman's blood pressure drops, the blood supply to her baby drops as well, with subsequently less oxygen reaching her baby.

To prevent low blood pressure, doctors load mothers up on IV fluid, prior to starting the epidural, to hopefully counteract the epidural's hypotensive effects.

Difficulty Urinating

When a woman receives an epidural, she typically does not have any feeling below its insertion point. About 15%[87] of women who receive an epidural will have difficulty urinating due to decreased bladder sensation. If this happens, they will have their bladder drained via a catheter inserted into their urethra. This is because a full bladder can impede labor progression. After the birth they may need to be catheterized as well, as a full bladder can cause very uncomfortable uterine cramps. Bladder sensation usually returns within a few hours after birth.

Itchy Skin

The medication administered through an epidural catheter can cause a side effect of an itchy sensation[88] all over the woman's body. While it can be very uncomfortable, it usually subsides within a few hours to a few days after birth.

Epidural Headache

When the anesthesiologist inserts the needle into a woman's back, if it penetrates just a few millimeters too deep past the epidural space, it may puncture the dura and cause cerebrospinal fluid to leak out. This is called a "wet tap."

Cerebrospinal fluid runs along the spine and surrounds and cushions the brain. The leak of cerebrospinal fluid causes a drop in the amount of cerebrospinal fluid in the brain, leading to a "post-dural puncture headache." Lying down relieves the headache, while sitting or standing up causes severe pain. Spinal headaches, also known as epidural headaches, are really uncomfortable and can last from a few days to a few weeks. A wet tap occurs in about 1%[89] of women receiving an epidural, and the risk may increase depending on the skill level of the anesthesiologist. The more skilled the anesthesiologist, the lower your risk of a wet tap. The best fix for a wet tap is a "blood patch[90]." This is where the anesthesiologist draws a small amount of the patient's blood and injects it into the spot where the spinal fluid is leaking, so that it clots and stops up the leak. Some doctors may be hesitant to do a blood patch because of the small risk for infection. They may recommend other measures, such as drinking caffeinated beverages and resting.

Longer Labor

Epidurals slow down[91] labor. Usually, you will see the slow down occur during the second stage of labor, also known as the "pushing phase." In 2014, a study[92] published in *Obstetrics & Gynecology* compared the length of the pushing phase for women who did not have an epidural with women who had one. They found pushing lasted about an hour longer if they had an epidural. The second stage may be considered "prolonged" depending on the circumstances. If a woman receives an epidural and it is her first birth, pushing for more than three hours is considered a prolonged second stage. If she does not receive an epidural, then more than two hours is considered prolonged for a first-time mother.

For a woman who has had a prior birth and has an epidural, pushing for more than two hours is prolonged. If she does not receive an epidural, then pushing for more than one hour is considered prolonged.

These are typical hospital protocols, although some hospitals and obstetrical practices may agree to allow a woman to push for a longer period of time.

What happens when a mom reaches the end of her "allotted time" to push out her baby? Typically, her doctor will give her a diagnosis of "failure to progress," or "labor dystocia," and either perform an assisted vaginal birth or a c-section. An assisted vaginal delivery can happen in two ways. The first method is using forceps[93], which look like two salad spoons. These are inserted into the vagina to help bring the baby down. The other method is via vacuum extraction, where the doctor attaches a soft plastic suction cup to the baby's head and uses suction to assist the baby down. Both of these methods can cause trauma to the baby and to the perineum. Mom may need an episiotomy or suffer tearing to her vagina. The baby will likely end up with some bruising on their head and/or face from the tools.

Why can't moms have more time to push? Why is a long pushing phase a problem? Health care providers and hospitals are concerned because a long second stage[94] of labor has been linked with an increased risk of postpartum hemorrhage (PPH) and severe perineal lacerations.

Postpartum Hemorrhage

Postpartum hemorrhage is excessive bleeding after birth. When moms experience a lengthy labor in a hospital setting, typically, her doctor will up her IV Pitocin drip in order to try and speed things up. A 2014 study found a link between Pitocin administration and increased risk of postpartum hemorrhage[95]. Pitocin is synthetic oxytocin, which is the hormone that stimulates the uterus to contract. Pitocin does not act exactly like oxytocin though. While oxytocin is released into our blood stream in spurts, Pitocin is a steady drip through an IV. Pitocin causes longer and more intense contractions. This, in turn, produces a risk for PPH as it can desensitize receptors on the uterus. This desensitization impairs the uterus's ability to contract effectively after birth. Instead of the uterus contracting tightly after birth, which reduces the amount of bleeding from the placenta attachment site, the uterus remains flaccid, causing hemorrhaging. The risk for PPH is mitigated, ironically, by receiving IV Pitocin after birth.

Another effect of IV Pitocin is the added stress it puts on the baby. The baby's oxygen supply decreases during contractions. When contractions are more intense, the baby is under more stress and more likely to decompensate. In this scenario, the doctor would recommend a c-section due to fetal distress.

Perineal Lacerations

Perineal lacerations, or vaginal tears, are pretty common during childbirth. Most women who tear during birth will suffer minor lacerations.

The severity of the lacerations are classified as "degrees."

- A first-degree tear is a small tear that may or may not require a couple of stitches. There is usually little discomfort with a first-degree tear.
- A second-degree tear involves skin and muscle and will require several stitches.
- A third-degree tear involves skin and muscle around the anus. This involves a number of stitches and discomfort will last from a few weeks to up to several months.
- A fourth-degree tear involves the anal sphincter, which is several muscles that work together to give you the ability to control your bowel movements. If this sphincter is torn during birth, it may cause long-term problems in some women, including bowel incontinence, which is a loss of control of bowel movements.

Pelvic floor disorders have a strong correlation[96] with assisted vaginal deliveries and coached pushing.

In 2007 the *American Journal of Obstetrics & Gynecology* published a study[97] that showed an increased risk in severe lacerations in women who received an epidural during labor.

In 2011, *the Journal of Fetal and Maternal Medicine* published a study[98] that found that women allowed to push for longer than three hours had lower odds of third and fourth-degree tears and NICU admission for their babies, than women who had assisted vaginal deliveries.

When would interventions be necessary in case of a long pushing phase?

In cases of true obstructed labor, where the baby is malpositioned and cannot move down, a c-section is necessary. The midwife and doctor need to look at prolonged labor to determine if it is true obstructed labor, or the mom is just progressing slowly but within a normal range.

Freedom of Movement

How can you avoid perineal trauma during labor?

An important way to avoid perineal trauma is to avoid pushing in the lithotomy position. The lithotomy position is the position you assume for pelvic exams, where you are lying on your back with your legs apart. In 2015, a study[99] published in Sweden found that birthing in the lithotomy position is associated with an increased risk for a third-degree tear.

Birthing upright[100] has been found to reduce the incidence of perineal tears as well as significantly reduce pushing time. This is because the pelvic outlet is at its smallest when a woman is lying on her back. The pelvic outlet becomes wider when a woman is upright. Birthing upright also allows the baby to utilize gravity as it moves down, which helps moves labor along as well.

Why are doctors reluctant to allow women to birth their babies in an upright position?

Doctors are primarily taught to deliver women in the supine position, which is lying on your back. This may be because doctors can better visualize the baby as it emerges from the birth canal. A more optimal position than the supine position is the left side-lying position[101], which most doctors are comfortable with as well.

During labor, moving around freely is beneficial[102], as there is a lower incidence of perineal injuries when you are free to move into positions that feel right to you. If you need an epidural but still want freedom of movement, some hospitals offer the option of having a low dose epidural that does not completely numb your legs. They can also cut off or reduce the anesthetic during the pushing phase so that you can push more effectively.

There are different pushing methods you can use that will minimize perineal trauma. The coached pushing method favored by doctors looks like this: Once a woman's cervix is fully dilated, her legs are placed in stirrups, or alternatively, bent and held close to their body assisted by the nurse. The patient is told to take a deep breath and push as hard as they can to the count of ten. The doctor has the patient do this several times during the contraction. Coached pushing[103] can damage the nerves of the perineum from the intense pressure it induces.

A gentler way to push is called open glottis[104] spontaneous pushing. This is where a mom bears down while slowly breathing out. The pelvic floor stretches more slowly as the baby descends, with less risk of damage to the pelvic floor. In a study[105] done comparing coached pushing to open glottis pushing, there was less perineal trauma for women using open glottis pushing.

A third method is passive pushing. A review of studies[106] show that for a woman with an epidural, passive pushing decreases the amount of pushing time the woman has to do later. Passive pushing is where the uterus is contracting during the pushing phase without any bearing down action. Passive pushing can be done for up to two hours[107] after full dilation has occurred. Passive pushing[108] contains a lower risk of pelvic floor trauma for the mother and less stress on the baby.

Episiotomy

An episiotomy is a surgical cut a doctor will make to enlarge the vaginal opening for the baby. Doctors claim several benefits:[109] It expedites the baby's birth, the cut heals better than a tear, and it protects against pelvic floor disorders.

A Cochrane Review[110], published in February 2017 found that routine episiotomies do not reduce perineal trauma in women giving birth. In addition, some women tear along the episiotomy, which will then then leave them with a third or fourth-degree laceration.

Rarely, an episiotomy may be necessary to enlarge the vaginal opening in a situation where the baby needs to be born quickly, but an episiotomy should never be routine.

The hospital birth setting has many routines and protocols that may or may not be evidence-based. Knowing the routines you may encounter at the hospital will help you make an informed decision when deciding where to have your baby.

CHAPTER 5
Midwives

For a healthy woman with a low-risk pregnancy, studies show that birthing with a qualified midwife will give her a safer and more satisfying birth experience than birthing with a doctor. Many women choose a midwife to deliver their baby in the hospital for a more natural and supported birth in a medical setting.

A study[111] done in 2009 in British Columbia, Canada showed a lower incidence of c-sections, electronic fetal monitoring, episiotomies, and other interventions at a hospital birth attended by a midwife than one attended by a doctor. In this study, infant mortality rates were identical, with improved birth experience for moms.

A 2016 Cochrane Review[112] found that low-risk women giving birth in the hospital had fewer interventions and were overall more satisfied with midwifery-led care than obstetrician-led care.

In the United States, only about 8% of births are attended by a midwife. In other countries, for example in Holland and England, midwives are the first point of care for pregnant women. Renske Kuiper[113], a Dutch midwife, describes the maternity system in Holland, "Most women, about 80% of women, will start with a midwife, and it's only the women that already have, for example, high blood pressure, diabetes, or other pre-existing health conditions that will see an Obstetrician directly."

Anne Cobell[114], a British midwife, observes in an interview, "In the UK we are under the proviso that every single woman needs a midwife, and only some women will need a doctor. So it's not like in the United States, Australia, or other parts of the world where you would predominantly see a doctor. Here, everyone sees a midwife."

The midwifery profession is the backbone of maternity care in countries like Holland and England. A pregnant woman will see a midwife for maternity care and will only be referred to an obstetrician if it is medically indicated.

The midwifery model of care follows the origin of the word "midwife," which means "with woman," in Old English. Midwives establish a relationship with their patients based on respect for a woman's autonomy over her own body.

Compared to doctors, midwives take a more laid-back approach to childbirth, while vigilantly keeping an eye on the mother and baby for any signs of trouble. As long as the mother and baby are doing fine, midwives understand that allowing the process to unfold naturally leads to better maternal and fetal outcomes. Doctors, on the other hand, prefer to manage the process as much as possible by intervening and "helping" it along.

Women who birth with midwives receive personalized care. Midwives stay with women during labor and provide labor support. This gives them the opportunity to remain vigilant and spot any potential problems sooner. They will stay at your side, helping you manage your contractions and advising you on which positions to assume. They will even give you a back rub. You will rarely find an obstetrician giving a back massage or helping a woman labor comfortably. At best, they will ask a nurse to try and settle you.

Hannah Dahlen[115], professor of midwifery at Western Sydney University and home birth midwife, describes her evolution,

"Every journey is so utterly unique, and I'd say I've become such an experienced midwife that I now no longer focus on how it's going to be. Because I've learned that every woman can surprise you. And our job as midwives is to watch birth unfold. If it's unfolding in a way that's jeopardizing safety, our job is to step in, but not until then."

Prenatal care with a midwife is a different experience than prenatal care with an obstetrician.

Mrs. Y. Engel, CM[116] describes the midwife and patient relationship, "When the patient and midwife develop a relationship through prenatal care, the woman feels supported; she feels heard and understood. It becomes a personal relationship that is conducive to relaxing and allowing the process of birth to happen."

Midwives will hear you out when you question a routine test, and either explain to you why they feel it is necessary or help you explore other options. For example, between the sixth and seventh month of pregnancy, it is recommended for all pregnant women to be screened for gestational diabetes, as about 4% of women are diagnosed with diabetes during pregnancy. Gestational diabetes, which is high blood sugar during pregnancy, can cause complications, so doctors and midwives use a one-hour glucose challenge test to screen for it.

The way the test works is by drinking a special glucose drink called Glucola. You have to drink it within five minutes, and then have a blood test an hour later to check your glucose level. If your glucose level is above 140, you will need further testing.

Some women react negatively to the Glucola[117], either vomiting from it or just not feeling well for the rest of the day. Some of the ingredients in the drink are also questionably unhealthy, as it includes additives like food coloring and brominated vegetable oil.

It's important to test for diabetes, as untreated diabetes can have serious repercussions for mom and baby. With this in mind, it is still possible to make the test as comfortable as possible while maintaining its accuracy. You'll find midwives are generally open to alternatives to Glucola. For example, you can consume 1 and ¼ cups of grape juice or apple juice or 28 jelly beans. These alternatives contain 50 grams of sugar which is the same as Glucola. As long as you consume 50 grams of sugar within 5 minutes, it is sufficient for the test. Many doctors, unfortunately, will not give you the option of consuming one of the above options, and will instead specifically require Glucola to be consumed for this test.

It is the idea of being mom-centered that differentiates the way a midwife practices to the way an obstetrician practices.

The book, *The Power of Moments*[118], by Chip Heath and Dan Heath, describes how doctors and health care providers can change their focus from treating the patient, to finding out how the patient wants to be treated. Asking patients what treatment and care they are looking for will allow their health care provider to center their care around their wishes and desires.

The midwifery profession excels in this approach. Having your health care provider ask you what your birth plan is, and what they can do to help you achieve it, will differentiate your birth experience. It is worth your while to seek out a health care provider who will do this for you.

Doctors generally view themselves as in charge, telling moms what they need to do to have their baby. Midwives[119] view their role as an advisor to the mother, explaining everything to her and educating her on what is happening to her and her baby. They are there to support mom as her pregnancy progresses and during birth.

Jennifer Griffin[120], home birth mom and author[121], credits her midwives with helping her learn to trust her own intuition.

> When I would say, "My stomach really hurts me here," they would respond, "Well what do you think it is?"
>
> And I was thinking, "What do you mean what do I think it is? What did I hire these people for?"
>
> And they would say, "Well, it could be this, this, this, or this. Some are potentially serious and some are nothing to worry about. So do you want to get another ultrasound?"
>
> I realized in the series of similar conversations that they were trying to empower me to take control of my care, which is pretty incredible.
>
> I know women who have gone into the hospital and have tried to speak up when they knew something was wrong and were ignored.
>
> The medical model is so fear-based and doctor dependent, and I talk in my recent book about how the midwives gave me my power back.

When asked what the most challenging part of having a home birth was, Jessica Cole[122], a home birth mom, shared in an interview:

> I think the biggest challenge was after the first couple of appointments with the midwife, realizing how empowered I was and that this was up to me to do.
>
> I was expecting more direction, but they were going to be taking direction from me. They were ready to do what came naturally to me during labor, and I think that responsibility made me realize that birthing my baby was up to me.

The midwifery model, as taught in midwifery school, is holistic, compared to the medical model obstetricians are taught. Midwives are strongly rooted in natural birth and empowering women through their pregnancy and birth experience.

Tamar van Haaren-ten Haken[123], professor and Dutch midwife, describes the maternity care structure in Holland:

"In the Netherlands, we always had a very strong vision separating births without complications from those with complications.

It was written into law in 1895 that normal birth should be done by midwives, and birth with complications should be done by medical doctors."

Tamar elaborates, "So in other countries, where there was no law supporting midwives, I think a lot of births were done in the end by doctors and hospitals, whereas we had the law on our side that we should care for women without any complications."

Renske Kuiper[124], a Dutch midwife, explains:

> In Holland, in order to become a midwife, the education is four years. It is separate from medicine or any medical education, so it's really a four-year education that is directly to become a midwife which covers all the aspects of a normal pregnancy, including delivery and postpartum period, and an abnormal pregnancy. You're trained to be the guard at the door, to say, "Okay, this is normal, this is not normal," and when to refer to the obstetrician.
>
> We have a good system where you have to be registered under BIG[1] in order to practice midwifery. So it's not like anyone can call themselves a midwife. You can only practice if you are registered and fulfilled all the education requirements.

---

1   "BIG: Beroepen in de Individuele Gezondheidszorg, professions in individual health care, registered by law, all professions like doctors, pharmacists, physiotherapists, psychotherapists, dentists and midwives are BIG registered)."

Mrs. Y. Engel, CM[125], a home birth midwife in New York, discusses obstetric and midwifery care:

> I am a big proponent of good doctors. We need doctors to take care of women when there is a problem. But we also need to be humble enough to recognize that pregnancy is a healthy stage in a woman's life. It's not a disease. We need to be able to recognize that. Midwives are keeping women healthy and safe, and good midwives will want to work collaboratively with good doctors. Ideally there has to be a relationship. When a midwife picks up something, she shouldn't think that she knows it all. She should refer and collaborate with a doctor, and when a doctor sees that a woman is healthy, he should be able to say, "You might do better with a midwife."

Ideally, obstetricians and midwives work together in a way that inspires trust in each other. Obstetricians and midwives both have their specialties, with midwives specializing in low-risk births and obstetricians specializing in high-risk, more medically complex births.

Helen Robinson, British midwife, states, "It's called 'shared care.' If something turns up and I don't think the woman needs to see the obstetrician, I'll book her into the clinic if I've got a particular concern, and I will email the obstetrician and discuss things together, so it's a good collaboration."

Trusting each other's expertise benefits pregnant women. When a midwife trusts a doctor it means she will ask questions as they come up and will refer as needed. Discussing their patient's care and exchanging thoughts leads to better outcomes for the mother and baby. When an obstetrician trusts the midwife, it means the obstetrician really listens to what the midwife is saying, which results in a smoother and more complete transfer of care. It inspires confidence in pregnant women that they are receiving good care and brings peace of mind that is so important for a pregnant woman to have.

Midwives have different routes to obtaining their certification, depending on the country they live in.

In the United States, there are several classes of midwives currently practicing.

A Certified Nurse Midwife (CNM) is a registered nurse with a master's degree in midwifery. Becoming a CNM includes studying for a four-year undergraduate nursing degree, and then an additional 2 years of study for a master's specializing in midwifery. After that is an orientation period during which she is supervised by an experienced midwife before practicing on her own.

A Direct-Entry Midwife (DEM[126]) is a midwife without a nursing degree. Direct-entry midwives include several subcategories, reflecting the state they are practicing in, and their legal designation. Examples of direct-entry midwives are Certified Professional Midwife (CPM[127]) and Licensed Midwives (LM). CPMs are certified nationally by the North American Registry of Midwives[128] (NARM). LMs are certified by the state the midwife practices in.

Direct-entry midwives do not have a college degree, but follow a specific course of study. For example, NARM requires the clinical component of the educational process to be at least 2 years in duration, and include a minimum of 55 births in 3 distinct categories. Clinical education must occur under the supervision of a midwife who is certified and legally recognized. The supervising midwife must have practiced for at least 3 years, and attended 50 out-of-hospital births post-certification. There is a written exam before CPM licensure.

A Certified Midwife CM[129] is a midwife with a master's degree in midwifery and is a health care professional but not a registered nurse. CMs are certified by Accreditation Commission for Midwifery Education (ACME[130]). A CM certification is only recognized in a handful of states in the United States.

The United States differs from other countries worldwide in that they have a variety of credentials for midwives. Almost every other country has only one path a person can take to becoming a midwife. For example, in Israel, a midwife has to be a Registered Nurse[131] with a four-year licensed nursing degree.

Barbara Ben Ami[132], Israeli midwife[133], describes the system in an interview:

> In Israel, midwives are only Nurse Midwives, what you call Certified Nurse Midwives (CNMs) in the United States. There are no CPMs (Certified Practical Midwives) here, only Nurse Midwives.
>
> Our scope of practice is less than in the US. For example, I cannot give referrals to the HMOs; they have to go to a doctor for that. I can't write prescriptions…
>
> You have to go to a university nursing school for a BSN. The midwifery course is given by the Ministry of Health in different hospitals in the country. The course is a little longer than one academic year. It's also a separate licensure. I have a license as a registered nurse, and I have a separate license as a midwife, but you can't have a license as a midwife without having a license as a nurse. According to the Ministry of Health, if you want to be a home birth midwife, you have to work for a minimum of three years in the hospital, for experience, etc., but there is no home birth midwife course. The problem with that is as a midwife in the hospital, you only work in the hospital delivery room. You don't do prenatals, you don't do postnatals, you don't

do well women checkups, like in America. You work in the delivery room period. That's all you do.

Here, women who use Israeli HMOs will see a doctor for their prenatal care. There might be a nurse there who takes their blood pressure and checks their urine, but the prenatal care is given by a doctor. Legally we're allowed to do prenatal care, but that's the way the system developed. So when I left the hospital and started becoming a home birth midwife, I had to learn all of this. I hadn't been doing proper prenatal care before, and I hadn't been doing postnatal care, so I had a lot to learn. I had to learn about jaundice and breastfeeding and newborn care, and how to suture. We didn't suture in the hospital. There were a lot of things I had to learn when I left the hospital.

It's more natural than in the US. Hospital births are not as medicalized as in the US. In the US, women have their doctor, he comes to do their birth, and it's a very medicalized birth; there is a very high cesarean section rate. The c-section rate, here in Israel, depends on the hospital. It's around 23% at most hospitals, but in some hospitals it's 30%. So we do have an overall lower c-section rate here.

When you go to the delivery room you are attended by whichever midwife is on call. You don't have your private midwife. It's more similar to socialized medicine. So when you come to the hospital, you have no idea who's going to be delivering your baby. You know it's a midwife and whoever you happen to fall on, if she's nice and you connect with her, that's great. If not, no. That's why a lot of women take doulas, because they want at least one familiar face to work with that they know.

Hannah Dahlen[134] describes the Australian birth system:

> In Australia we have a system probably halfway between the US and England. 25% of women have private insurance, which means that for their birth they have a private obstetrician who does their antenatal care and who comes in at the last moment to catch the baby; the midwives in the hospital do all the rest of the care.
>
> The other 75% are cared for in a variety of models. Around 10% of those women now are in continuity of midwifery care programs where they have a known midwife who provides antenatal care, comes in for their birth, and does postnatal care. That's 10% of women.
>
> The remaining 55-60% of women are cared for in a variety of fragmented models. There might be shared care with a general practitioner. There might be shared care between a midwife and a midwife clinic, where one midwife catches the baby and different midwives do the postnatal care. Or it might be that they have risk factors so they go to the doctor's clinic and midwives do the care and the birth.

Hannah describes midwifery regulations in Australia:

> We have one registration so whether you do your Bachelor of Midwifery degree, or whether you're a nurse that goes on to do 18 months of postgraduate midwifery, you come out with the same registration. Then we have codes of conduct, we have registration and education standards, we have to complete audits every year around whether or not there's been any notifications on your practice. There's a lot of requirements around regulating midwifery in Australia.

Countries around the world have different education requirements for licensed midwives, which is important to keep in mind when researching midwives in your area.

CHAPTER 6

How to Prepare for a Home Birth

C haya's Story[135]

I am sharing with you the birth of my fourth child. I had five home births. My oldest is 16 years old and my youngest is 20 months old.

Before I got pregnant with my fourth child I started using my current midwife who lives in my community. I was already visiting her for my regular woman's care, so I had already gotten to know her before I got pregnant this time around. I got in touch with her when I was about 9 weeks pregnant and went to visit her at the 12 week mark.

I went for my monthly prenatal visits and did all the necessary blood work, the 20 week sonogram, the 28 week sugar test, later blood tests, and all of the routine prenatal testing that is recommended for pregnant women.

The prenatal visits we would take between 45 minutes to an hour.

People often ask me "What do you do at your midwife's office for an hour? All you have to check is blood pressure, baby's heartbeat, size of baby, leave a urine sample in the bathroom. What takes that long?"

That's where everything changes with a home birth midwife. In addition to doing all the technical stuff, we discuss everything around the home birth, the pregnancy, any concerns, whether it's physical or emotional, familial, any type of planning, from prebirth to at the birth itself, and post birth. Since this went on at prenatal visits, by the time I got to the actual birth, there was a very comfortable relationship between us. We both knew what to expect from each other.

At week 36, my midwife and her assistant, who I had met twice before, came to visit me at my home. This was done so that they got to see what the drive is like and where exactly my home is. Prior to that appointment, the midwife gave us a list of things to prepare in our home, so she checked that everything from the list was indeed ready.

I continued with prenatal visits, and my midwife continued to monitor me to ensure I stayed healthy and low-risk. This is because a prerequisite for home birth is that the mom is low-risk. Low-risk means mom is otherwise healthy, there's no other health complications, and the pregnancy is progressing in a normal, healthy fashion. If there are any sugar issues or high blood pressure or other complications, that may become high-risk. At that point, there would be a conversation about possibly transferring to a hospital and whatever options there are.

For me, thankfully, everything moved along uneventfully. When I was 2 days past my due date, I went into labor. My three older children at the time were between ages 7 and 3, and I chose not to have them at home for the birth. Early in the evening, when I realized this might really be happening, we put them to sleep at a family member's home that we had planned beforehand.

I started to labor with just me and my husband at home. I called the midwife to notify her of what was going on, but I told her she does not need to come over yet since it was early and I was managing well. A woman who stays home doesn't need to worry about when to go to the hospital, if it's too early, too late, or any of those kinds of thoughts. I am very communicative with my midwife as to where I'm at and at what point I want her in my house.

A couple of hours later, around 11:00 p.m., when I felt the contractions much stronger and moving closer together, I called her again and told her to come over. She came with her assistant. At that point, I was laboring in the bathtub. I asked her to check where I was up to.

They listened to the baby, they checked that mom is doing well, baby is doing well, then they did a vaginal check and I was open 5 centimeters. Labor was still manageable, meaning that I was able to talk between contractions and rest between contractions, but they were becoming more intense.

A couple of hours later, I asked the midwife to check me again, and at that point I was only open 7 centimeters. For me, this was slow progress, and I was starting to get anxious. With my first three, things moved along quicker so I was starting to get nervous. "Why is this taking so long? Is everything okay?"

Baby sounded good and everything looked good, but because of my concerns the midwife decided to check vaginally to see and feel which position the baby was coming down in. She was able to feel, according to the way the head was, that the baby was coming down from a side angle, as opposed to straight down. In this case, the baby was not putting as much pressure down on the cervix with each contraction, and thereby making the labor much slower. This was something that was only picked up because we were both very in tune to the situation and into how I was feeling and how things were progressing.

At this time, we discussed what we could do to help the baby shift and help labor progress. We decided that I should not labor in the bathtub anymore and I should move into an upright position, with gravity helping the baby come down. We decided to go for a brisk walk.

It was late in the middle of the night, around 3 a.m., and I went with my husband brisk walking outside as well as inside my house, up and down the hallway, stopping every so often to breath through contractions. That helped the baby move into a better position.

A couple of hours later, I felt like labor progressed a lot. I felt my body was going through transition as I was experiencing a range of emotions, more tears, more crying, more shakiness, as well as closer together contractions. I couldn't talk or rest much between them. This told us that labor was progressing nicely.

A short while later, I was starting to feel the baby coming lower, and the sensation of pushing began. My midwife did not check me again; she trusted the way I felt and that I was getting ready to push. I don't really push my babies, I don't go into that "one-two-three push" situation. I wait to feel those strong, strong contractions, where the baby is starting to crown, and I bear down together with the contractions. I like to be in an upright position, where the gravity helps the baby be born. I was standing in my room, leaning over the dresser; it was just the perfect height, coming right up to my diaphragm. I was leaning over, bending my knees a little bit and working along with the contractions.

My midwife was kneeling right behind me to catch the baby. I felt that burning sensation of the baby crowning. Since I like to feel how my baby is born, I put my hand down to feel the head come out, and with another one of those contractions, the baby was born!

My midwife caught the baby and pushed it forward to me so that I could scoop it up and bring it to my chest skin-to-skin. I still didn't see what the baby was, boy or girl. The midwife supported me under my arm. I had to take a couple of steps back to my bed, holding my baby, who had started to cry. I sat down with my baby on me and then laid down to my side. At that point I picked up the baby, moved it to see what it was, and sure enough it was a boy. Our first boy after three girls! It was the most beautiful sight!

After about 15 minutes, the placenta came out. My midwife then gave us our privacy so we could bond with our baby. The baby lay on my chest and started to root, looking to suck, and then he began nursing.

In that hour, the midwife and her assistant cleaned up the room, putting things into the garbage, and popped a couple of things into the washing machine. They did it so quickly, without any noise, and the room was clean and fresh.

They checked me as well in that hour to make sure the bleeding was okay and that there was no laceration (tear), which there wasn't. After an hour, they did the baby assessment, checking his weight and size.

Approximately 3 hours after the baby was born and everything was settled, we were doing well. Baby had fed and they helped me dress him. I showered and freshened up. My husband was with me. Everything looked nice and calm at that point. The midwives then left.

They came back at the 24 hour mark, 5 days, 2 weeks, and then we scheduled a 6 week postpartum visit in the office. They were available at any time if I had any question or any concern. I did have a lactation issue with this baby as he had tongue tie which needed to be fixed. Any little thing that came up, they were there available for me, night or day.

Thanks to such a wonderful experience, we were so happy and calm and were able to just enjoy the pleasures of a new baby in the house. The girls came home to meet their brother and bond as a new family.

What does planning a home birth entail? How do you prepare for it? The weeks before your due date will be full of preparations. Your midwife will give you a list of things to gather, as well as a home birth kit to purchase online. Most home birth midwives have a personal online kit that is already assembled by the company. She will give you a link to purchase it online and have it shipped straight to your door.

What's in a home birth kit?

Each midwife has their own preferences for their home birth kits. Below is a typical one, which costs around $120.

6 disposable under-pads, size 30x30

2 Depends style disposable underpants

3 contour pads

1 peri bottle

2 mesh pants

1 Instant Perineal Cold Pack, which is soothing after birth and reduces perineal swelling

1 Delee 8fr suction trap

2 Tenderfoot lancets for newborn testing

2 newborn hats, one cotton

2 flex straws for drinking during labor. It helps to have a straw in the glass so you don't have to physically lift it while you're laboring.

1 paper tape measure to measure the baby's length at birth

2 plastic umbilical clamps to clamp the umbilical cord at birth

10 non-sterile disposable gloves

20 sterile gloves

3 surgical sterile gloves

1 Neet Feet Footprinter to capture baby's foot prints

10 alcohol prep pads

15 packets of lubricating jelly

1 pint of Isopropyl Alcohol (rubbing alcohol)

1 pint hydrogen peroxide

1 bulb syringe to clear baby's nose and mouth at birth

2 4x4 sterile gauze, trays of 10

1 rectangular basin

1 Amnicot/amnihook in case water needs to be broken

1 urethral catheter kit in case mom can't pass urine

2 IV administration sets in case of emergency

2 IV start kits

2 IV catheters, 22g

2 suture, 3.0 Vicryl GS21, in case mom needs stitches after birth

1 AmnioTest in case mom is not sure if her water broke. This test will check to see if fluid leaking out is amniotic fluid.

1 6cc syringe with 22g x 1 ½ needle

1 3cc syringe with needle

1 1cc syringe with needle

Some midwives bring their own IV kits and catheters, so you don't have to order them. Most women at a home birth won't actually need them.

The home birth kit should be ordered between weeks 35 and 36 of pregnancy as it'll take several days to come.

In addition to the home birth kit, there is another list of items to assemble:

6 bath towels that you don't mind throwing out after the birth

2-4 vinyl-backed tablecloths or shower curtains to protect your floor and bed

6 receiving blankets for baby

2 flashlights with extra batteries

1 package of newborn diapers

2 or more onesies and sleepers to dress baby in

1 roll of paper towels

1 digital thermometer

1 package of pads

2 yard-sized garbage bags and 1 kitchen-sized garbage bag

Ibuprofen for postpartum pain

What does your midwife bring?

Your midwife will bring emergency equipment, including an oxygen tank with masks for mom and baby, pulse oximeter to check your baby's oxygen saturation and heart rate, newborn resuscitation equipment, and a scale to weigh your baby.

A midwife also has on hand the vitamin k injection and erythromycin eye ointment for your baby, as per standard recommended practice. The vitamin k[136] injection prevents vitamin k deficiency bleeding, which is a rare but potentially fatal disease in newborns. Erythromycin eye ointment[137] prevents ophthalmia neonatorum, a serious eye infection. It is caused by gonorrhea or chlamydia bacterial infection, which are sexually transmitted diseases (STDs). It can be picked up by the baby if the bacteria are present in the vaginal canal. The pros and cons of giving these medications can be discussed with your health care provider.

"In the hospital, labor and delivery is led by the doctors and nurses. At a birthing center, the birth is midwife led. At home, it is woman led," shares Leah Marinelli,[138]a home birth midwife.

When you give birth at home you have the luxury of choosing whatever equipment you wish, and for many home birth moms that includes a birthing tub.

Many women enjoy sitting in a birthing tub during labor. Water exerts a counter pressure to the contractions, which makes them more manageable. Relaxing your body makes labor progress at a faster pace.

Some women will remain in the water for a water birth[139]. A 2004 study[140] published in the *Journal of Perinatal Medicine* found that mothers who had a water birth suffered less blood loss and had a lower rate of NICU admissions for their babies than women who birthed their babies out of the water.

In a 2009 study[141] of water birth in Iran, 106 women were randomly assigned to either a water birth or conventional delivery, and a questionnaire was completed by both groups of women. The study found that the women who had a water birth had no negative effects for themselves or their babies. They also requested less pain medication, and significantly, the active phase and third stage of their labor was shorter by an average of 72 minutes.

Water birth is safe under the guidance of a midwife or doctor, and mothers may be screened prior to birth for any infections that may be transferred to baby through the water.

When a baby is born in a water birth[142], they are lifted up to the surface to take their first breath while the rest of their body remains in the warm water. Water birth is very soothing and calming for a new baby, as well as their mother.

Some local hospitals have a birthing tub available for women to use while in labor, although you will want to ascertain if they are permitted for both water immersion during labor as well as water birth. Some hospitals do not permit the baby to be born in the water, and will ask you to step out for the birth.

A birthing tub is a lot bigger than your standard bathtub, so women choosing a home birth may want to purchase one. You can buy one online, or you may be able to rent or borrow one from your midwife. If you rent or borrow a birthing tub, you will need to purchase a tub liner. You will also need a clean hose and a hose adaptor in order to attach it to your faucet, as well as an automatic pump to blow it up. Be sure to have a practice run filling it up, as you don't want to find out while you're in labor that the hose doesn't fit right, or that you ran out of water, or that there's a tear and it leaks.

To protect your floor from drips and spills when getting in and out of the tub, lay down a blanket for padding on the floor, then place a vinyl-backed tablecloth or shower curtain on top of it, with the tub on top. You may also want to lay down a waterproof drop cloth walkway to your bathroom. You can pick up a drop cloth at a painting supply hardware store.

If birthing your baby in your bed is a possibility, you should take steps to protect your mattress.

Start off by covering it with a shower curtain or a waterproof mattress cover fitted on top of clean sheets. You can lay additional sheets over the waterproof barrier that you don't mind tossing after the birth. This way, after you get cleaned up, your midwife or doula can just roll everything up in the shower curtain and you'll have a nice clean bed to snuggle with your baby in.

Prepare your pillow by putting a clean pillowcase on it, then place it inside a garbage bag and cover it with another pillowcase you don't mind throwing out. Do that with several pillows.

The "Doing It At Home" podcast, found at www.diahpodcast.com, is a great resource for everything home birth. In Episode 141,[143] Matthew and Sarah Bivens, the podcast's hosts, share tips covering the gamut of things you may need or want to have at a home birth.

Matthew and Sarah recommend having a really well-stocked fridge in the days leading up to your due date. You might want to have Gatorade, water bottles, fresh fruit and vegetables, juice, milk, bread, pasta, and some of your favorite snacks. You'll want to have some snacks for your labor support people, too. You may also want to cook and freeze some meals in your freezer.

Flameless candles provide a warm ambience, and a playlist of your favorite songs gets you in the zone. Music during labor reduces pain perception, and will calm and relax you. Studies[144] show that listening to music during labor reduces labor pain and anxiety, as well as reduces the need for pain medication.

Drawing or printing birth affirmations on cards to hang up on the wall provides a focus for your mind in the weeks leading up to labor. Birth affirmations creates a positive mindset that empowers you for birth.

Examples of birth affirmations:

"I've got this."

"My strong, powerful body knows what to do."

"Each contraction is a gift as it brings my baby down into my arms."

"My mind quiets. My body opens."

"Each contraction is like a strong ocean wave. I let it wash over me as my baby moves down."

"I relax through each contraction as I open up for my baby."

"The slower you breathe, the calmer you feel."

You can find them on Etsy as beautiful printables.

Affirmations are incredibly strong messages you send to your brain. Sending your mind positive messages before and during birth will impact your birth, as well as frame your perception of your baby's birth. Viewing yourself as strong and seeing your contractions as a sign of your strength, will empower you to flow with the contractions instead of against them. Your mind influences your body in a very powerful way, and conditioning your mind prior to birth can really impact your experience.

Hypnobirthing[145] is a program that helps you work with affirmations to get into a zone where you are able to use your mind to refocus on relaxing your body through the contractions, instead of tensing up. Hypnobirthing teaches you to hypnotize yourself into a state of deep mental and physical relaxation using deep breathing, visualizations, and affirmations. Hypnobirthing participants reframe contractions as "waves" or "surges," and welcome them as they come. This method advocates free and unrestricted movement during labor, dedicated labor support, and no routine medical interventions. Practicing hypnobirthing techniques in the weeks leading up to your baby's birth is key. That way your mind can slip right into it when you need it.

Sarah Lewis[146], a home birth mom, shared in an interview about birth, "I really feel like being in labor and giving birth is mind over matter. You have to have total confidence in your body that this is what your body was designed to do. The same way people can endure physical feats and just put their mind above the physical pain and focus on the end goal; every contraction is bringing you closer to your baby, so it is actually exciting.

It's painful, but it's not useless or pointless. It is purposeful pain."

When a runner is speeding down the track, his pumping leg muscles cause an endorphin release called a "runner's high." The endorphin release is that wonderful feeling you have after a really good workout. Your uterus is getting a really good workout during labor, and endorphins[147] are released in response. These endorphins help a woman in labor get into a zone where she doesn't feel the passage of time in the same way. Endorphins helps moms manage the intensity of the contractions as endorphin[148] levels increase as contractions intensify. It is really a marvel how your body knows what to do to birth your baby.

Planning for your birth and thinking about what you would like to have available to help you manage your contractions is important. It's also hard to know what will work for you during labor, so it is a good idea to prepare several ideas and things that may help you during labor.

The following story told by Barbara Ben Ami[149], an Israeli home birth midwife, is a great example of how unpredictable circumstances around birth are, and how you have to work with what you have.

> I once had this woman, it was her second birth, she was living in an apartment building in one of the more poorer sides of the city, and she was in the shower the whole time. She really felt good with the water.
>
> Suddenly, somebody shut off the water in the building, and she says to her husband, "What's going on? I need the water."
>
> So he went downstairs and sees there's a plumber working on the water system to the building. I can hear them through the window in the bathroom on the fourth floor. He went down the four flights of stairs and I hear him

saying to the plumber, "Turn on the water, turn on the water, my wife is giving birth."

And the plumber's like, "What do you mean your wife is giving birth?"

"My wife's giving birth, we need the water, turn the water on."

And the plumber said, "If your wife's giving birth, why don't you go to the hospital?"

He said, "No, we're having a home birth."

So he says, "What do you mean you're having a home birth?"

So he says, "I can't talk, just please turn the water on."

And he goes, "Okay, okay I'll turn the water on. Ask your wife when she's going to have the baby because I have to finish this. It's Friday and I have to finish before Shabbat (Sabbath)."

And I'm up there cracking up because I can hear all this through the window. So the guy comes running up four flights of stairs and he said, "Ok, the water's back on, the guy wants to know when you're going to give birth."

I looked at him, like "Really?" and said, "Tell them an hour and a half."

So he goes running down the flight of stairs and I hear him telling the guy, "An hour and a half."

The guy says, "Okay, okay I'll wait an hour and a half."

There is a group of these old Moroccan ladies sitting downstairs talking in the garden, having tea. This woman was very, very vocal. At the end, she's in the shower, and she's getting really loud, and she makes a lot of noise, and then the baby's born. And the baby starts to cry. And suddenly we hear from downstairs in the garden, all of these old ladies whooping, "Mazel Tov!" These women are cheering, four or five old ladies cheering. And the girl is sitting there on my birth stool in the shower and holding her baby.

She looks and me and says, "See, that's why I wanted to have a home birth. It's private, it's intimate, it's in my home, nobody's there, just me and my husband and you...and the whole neighborhood!"

CHAPTER 7

Who Should You Invite to Your Home Birth?

W ho you choose to invite to your home birth is entirely up to you. You can keep it cozy with just your partner, your midwife, and her assistant, or you could turn it into a party of ten people or more. However you do it, the only thing that matters is that the people who are there are there because you want them there.

If you are looking into having additional people at birth to assist you, the first person I would look into having is a birth doula. A birth doula is a specially trained birth professional who supports a woman during labor and birth, as well as during the immediate postpartum period. Doulas can make all the difference between a positive and negative birth experience.

A 2017 Cochrane Review[150] study showed that women who received continuous one-on-one support throughout labor had shorter labors, fewer medical interventions, improved birth outcomes, higher Apgar scores, and increased satisfaction with their birth experience.

Doulas are birth specialists. They pull all the pieces of planning your birth together. They have studied and experienced birth to the extent that they intuitively recognize what will help. They will suggest position changes to keep labor from stalling. They know how to get you comfortable. They will look you in the eye and breathe through the contraction with you. They will remind you of your birth plan wishes when decisions need to be made. They will support your choices and advocate for you whether it's to your midwife, your doctor, or the nurses in the hospital. After the birth, a doula facilitates bonding and helps you and your baby begin your breastfeeding journey.

A doula will provide you with informational support. When your doctor or midwife tells you something is going on, your doula will help you understand the issue and how it will affect you. They will help you make the decision that is right for you.

When you plan for birth there are so many variables that will affect how it plays out. Every labor is different, and you just can't predict its course. It is impossible to know how long your labor will be, especially with a first birth, so knowing you have a doula on hand can bring you peace of mind. A doula will give your midwife and partner a rest. Your doula will provide direction to your birth partner, giving them tips and ideas on how to help you best. She makes it possible for them to catch a break and grab something to eat or drink. Your midwife needs to be clear-headed for the birth, so having someone dedicated for labor support can make a big difference.

How do you pick out a doula?

You will want to interview several doulas in your community, as well as hear about other women's experiences with them. Doulas differ in their philosophies and approach to childbirth, and you want your ideologies to align. Just like you choose a midwife or doctor who shares your vision for birth, you and your doula need to be a good fit as well.

For example, some doulas will do everything possible to ensure their moms do not get an epidural, while others feel there is a time and place for them.

You will also want to find out how much experience she has and what her go-to ideas are during labor. It is also important to call references to get some insight into her style and practices.

A doula will offer you at least one meeting prior to your birth to discuss your birth plan[151]. A birth plan is a way for you to systematically review your options for childbirth and make the decisions with your partner and doula regarding your preferences. It is not written in stone, and you can always change your mind while in labor. A birth plan clarifies your wishes and gives your doula an understanding of what you will want from her during labor.

Your birth plan should include things that will relax you during labor, such as back massages, foot rubs, dim lights, a shower, birthing tub, essential oils, and soft music.

You will also want to state your preference on having an epidural or other pain medication.

For a hospital birth, a doula plays an even more critical role. Your doula will do the following:

- Keep curtains closed around your bed to ensure your privacy
- Turn the light back off after your doctor or midwife leaves the room

- Advocate for you when your doctor wants to do an intervention and help you make the decision that's right for you
- Keep you informed of what's happening and remind you of your options
- Advocate for you if your epidural is wearing off
- Put a bucket in front of you if you need to throw up
- Keep your environment and everyone around you calm
- Alert your midwife or doctor when you feel an urge to push
- If an intervention is taking place without your knowledge, the doula will alert you and give you the space to verbalize your consent or refusal
- If you are not able to engage with hospital staff at a point during labor, your doula can be your voice

Your doula will be available for you when labor begins, and will come over to your home to help you labor. They will communicate with your midwife or doctor and describe where you are up to in labor. If you are planning a hospital birth, they will recognize when it is time to go to the hospital, and they will let your midwife or doctor know and then accompany you in the car.

Once your baby is born, your doula will stay with you for several hours after birth. She will facilitate breastfeeding, advocate for you and your baby, and ensure you have the space you need to bond with your baby.

Some doulas will stop by a day or two after birth to check in on you and see how you're doing. You can discuss your feelings about the birth, and she will help you understand what happened at the birth and why.

Many doulas are committed to helping every pregnant woman who wants a doula at their birth have one. Doulas do what they do because they love it and relish the privilege of helping a mom birth her baby. If cost is an issue, many doulas will work with you to help make their service affordable. You may be recommended to doulas-in-training who would love the experience and may be available to you at no cost. You can also add doula services to your wish list for your baby registry, and a friend or family member can gift it to you.

You may also have a friend or family member who you feel would be better than any doula out there, and they can be your doula.

Ruthie[152], a doula herself, has a fun birth story illustrating how having other support people at your birth can be really helpful.

Ruthie's Story

Around dinner time, I went to Leah's house to get checked and I was still 1 centimeter. I remember eating dinner with her and talking and getting more serious contractions. Then I was pacing her house pretty hard-core for the 35 seconds that they lasted. They weren't so close together. They were about 10 minutes apart. When I came home, my kids had been put to bed and then my contractions started picking up. At one point I was like, "Oh, I think this is actually it."

At this time Lauren had a patient in the hospital who had ruptured membranes (meaning their water broke), and in case she had to leave, she brought in Billy, RN and doula, Chiropractor Suzy, Mom, my niece, my sister-in-law, and her best friend who's a doula, Leah the midwife, and her daughter, Ilana, because we had been doula training together. Two of Lauren's daughters, Yael and Nechama, came as well, as I had been working in their house for the past couple of years and I was a part of the family. My good friend Devorah, who had always wanted to experience a birth, was there at my house having put my kids to bed for me, so she was there as well. So there were 11 of us along with my husband. My dad was downstairs. My kids were in the next room sleeping.

I spent some time in the tub, and the chiropractor did great counter-pressure. I felt zero pain during those contractions. When I started hyperventilating, I

got out and I remember walking with my big belly from the tub to my bed with
everyone standing and watching, and I was like, "We should sing kumbaya."
Then I reached a point...

Lauren said: "The baby's not in the best position," and Billy suggested doing
a Trochanter Roll[53], which is a prop under the hip in a certain place that is
super uncomfortable and uncomfortable for the baby as well. It caused him to
flip to the right side.

Once that happened Lauren sent everyone out of the room so I wouldn't be
distracted and I could focus and be at peace, and my husband and I could have
some time...

My baby was born at 1:31 a.m.

I remember that once he was born, Lauren told me after it was a lot like her
daughter having a baby, as I had been working at her house for 2 years, and
it was a special thing for us.

Lauren left sooner than she would have as she had a patient in the hospital.
Everyone left by 3:30, and we snuggled and lounged, enjoying our new baby.

At 5:30, my mother-in-law called to find out what was happening, so we
spent some time sharing our happy news. By the time we finished that phone
call, we woke up the kids. "Hey come meet your new brother."

Cool thing about a home birth is we conceived our baby in this room, we had
our baby in this room, and his name came to us in this same room.

Ruthie had many people at her home birth, including a chiropractor[154]. A chiropractor is a medical professional who makes adjustments to a person's spine using their hands or an instrument in order to improve spinal motion. The adjustments a chiropractor makes will help your body function optimally. Chiropractors focus on musculoskeletal disorders, lower back pain, sports injuries, migraines, as well as many other disorders. In addition, chiropractors successfully treat many pregnancy aches and pains.

When a chiropractor adjusts a pregnant woman and realigns her spine and hips, her baby will have more room to maneuver during birth. This follows the theory that if your body is in alignment, your baby will shift into an optimal position for birth.

After birth, moms may benefit from further chiropractic adjustments to establish pelvic balance and correct any misalignments that may have occurred during childbirth.

A chiropractor is a great addition to your birth team. Just verify the chiropractor you choose has experience working on pregnant women.

Jennifer Griffin[155], a home birth mom, shares her story in an interview:

> My four births were all the same, 18 hours long. Three started at night between 10 and midnight. The first time, the midwives came early, and I was scared and anxious, so they stayed up with me that whole night.
>
> With my second and third births, they came in the morning and so one would come first and stay with me and help with labor support and then the second midwife would join closer to the birth.
>
> I had back labor with all of them, which was really intense. I used acupuncture during pregnancy and with my last three births, my acupuncturist came to my birth. She actually asked to come!
>
> She came and treated me while I was laboring, and it really helped relieve the back pain. It was so amazing.

Jennifer had an acupuncturist at her home birth. Acupuncture is a method of placing hair-thin needles on specific locations throughout the body in order to target pathways to body. Acupuncture has grown more popular recently due to its benefits. It helps with chronic pain, migraines, mental health, gastro-intestinal problems, and infertility, among many other health issues.

Women have also found acupuncture helps ease pregnancy ailments as well as prepares their bodies for childbirth by ripening the cervix and facilitating cervical dilatation. During labor, research[156] shows acupuncture may significantly reduce pain and duration of labor.

Acupressure is a similar idea to acupuncture in that it revolves around specific points on the body, but instead of inserting needles, the practitioner applies manual pressure. Additionally, women have found that acupressure[157] has helped jump start their labor, as well as restart stalled labor. It strengthens contractions and eases the intensity of contractions.

The benefits are similar to acupuncture, but research shows that while acupuncture helps with cervical ripening, softening and effacing, acupressure does not help with those symptoms.

It is possible for your partner to learn how to apply accupressure during labor, as you just need to know where to apply pressure. You can use your fingers, knuckles, or even your elbows to apply acupressure. If your partner is unsure about it, you can ask your acupressure practitioner if they would like to attend your birth. You may be pleasantly surprised by their positive response.

A masseuse, also known as a massage therapist, can really help you relax during labor, as well as ease back labor. Different techniques that may make a difference include hip squeezes or lower back counter-pressure. You can also ask your doula or birth partner to give you a back rub or apply counter-pressure.

A birth photographer and/or videographer is a nice addition to your birth team. You can also just ask a friend to be there to snap photos or video of those special moments.

Some couples include their children in their home birth. The decision to include your children is a very personal one, and will greatly depend on your child's personality and abilities. The person who can best predict how your child will handle the birth experience is you. It's your child, and you've seen them in different situations and know best how they are likely to react. Some kids respond so well and love being able to help and be a part of the magic of birth. On the other hand, some children may not be able to participate in the capacity of "helper," either because they feel uncomfortable with what's going on, or they just get bored. If you choose to have your child present, make sure to designate an adult to be responsible for your child. That way they can redirect them in another room in the house or take them out for a drive.

April Davis[158], a home birth mom, envisioned having her children present at her baby's birth, but it didn't go as planned.

> My daughters were 7 and 4 at the time, and I was planning on having them there.
>
> We did a lot of prep work when I was pregnant, explaining everything about birth. I felt both my children were really well-prepared to be there to be a part of it.
>
> My sister came over right before I delivered, assumed I was in early labor, and took my girls to go to the store, and they ended up missing the birth. I'm still kind of devastated about it.
>
> They were okay with it, and my doula did everything she could to help incorporate them in my care, so they felt like they were there.
>
> They helped weigh him and measure him.
>
> I loved that. I like that they were part of the process, that they got to see that birth is such a normal event, and that I was fine.

It's good to gauge how your kids are going to be beforehand and plan accordingly, as not all kids will react the same way. I've been to some home births where the kids sleep through everything, and when they wake up in the morning, they get to meet the new baby.

Sarah Lewis[159], already with two little kids, describes her third birth which took place at home:

> My third home birth was right before a bad snowstorm hit, and I had two little kids at home. At the time, my parents were a few hours away, and I was just so relieved that I was having the baby at home and not having to go out to the hospital in a snowstorm and have to find childcare for my other kids. I just felt that having my kids at home with me while having my baby at home was a big relief and comfort.

You can prepare your child for birth by describing for them who will be there and the different things Mommy will do while in labor. It is also nice to involve them in prenatal appointments. Most midwifery practices are kid-friendly and have toys for kids to play with in the waiting room.

It may be helpful to have an older child around, just in case. Shoshana Levy[160] relates her home birth story:

> It started when I went into labor at 5 o'clock in the morning. I was focused on dealing with contractions, so I wasn't really timing them too much. This was with my second husband, and it was his first home birth experience, so he was nervous about the whole thing, and he left it to me to know what to do.
>
> I was doing so nicely by myself that I didn't realize how close things were getting, so I didn't tell him to call the midwife soon enough.

By 11 o'clock, I was hanging out in my bedroom in the rocking chair, and at one point told my husband, "I kind of feel like I have to push. You better call the midwife."

It happens to be my midwife lives really close, only about 5 minutes from my house. I didn't want to bother her too early, and I just did it on my own. I was doing hypnobirthing, so I was just chilling during the contractions getting my thoughts inside.

The most beautiful thing, I don't have to tell you, was that you're in your house, nobody's messing with you, nobody's telling you what to do, nobody's disturbing your peace.

When my midwife, Leah, came, she was racing and just ripping her packages open, yelling, "Get on the bed, get on the bed."

I was like, "Yeah, I kind of feel like I have to push."

So I got on the bed and she was like, "Yeah I see the baby's head!" and 2 pushes later she was out.

My 15-year-old daughter had to help out as Leah's assistant didn't have time to get here because she lives further away, so my 15-year-old was there handing Leah her gloves and holding the flashlight.

She actually got to cut the baby's cord.

I was able to relax in my bed and then take a shower in my own bathroom afterwards which was really nice.

I was amazed at how strong and capable I turned out to be.

I would never ever know my own strength.

The wellspring of feminine power is awesome.

It is an awesome thing which people are not allowed to experience.

They literally terrorize you with interventions and fear.

It's incredible when you leave a woman alone what she's capable of doing.

It's so empowering and it's just stunning.

So I think that the most beautiful thing about a home birth is that it lets a woman have an experience that even in the best hospital birth you're not going to fully get what it could have been if you were really left to your own devices, except for the minimum amount of support that you need to be safe.

It's something that's lost today.

Most women think you need all kinds of equipment and medical care when having a baby, but they're being cheated out of an incredible empowering experience and they don't know it.

CHAPTER 8

What Exactly Can Go Wrong During Birth?

Leah Marinelli[161], CNM, relates what happens when a pregnant mom comes to see her requesting a home birth:

> When someone comes to interview me for a home birth, I give them a consent form and we go through all the pros and cons.
>
> I explain the different emergencies that can happen which, although rare, may end up with more poor outcomes if they happen at home rather than in a hospital.
>
> There are cases where a NICU or surgery are needed right away, and while they are rare, when they happen, they need to be dealt with as quickly as possible.

Hospital birth provides women with medical conditions, or pregnancy complications the opportunity to have healthy babies. For some women with low-risk pregnancies, a hospital birth gives them the peace of mind of knowing an operating room and perinatal team are available just 30 seconds away, in case of an emergency.

If there was an emergency at a home birth, it would take some time to get to the hospital. That remains the determining factor for many women who choose to give birth at the hospital. The security of having obstetricians and an operating room on stand-by, is very reassuring. Most hospitals have neonatologists available as well, in case of a birth emergency. A neonatologist specializes in providing care in complex and high-risk situations. If a baby is born with a congenital disorder, such as a heart defect, they can provide rapid specialized neonatal support.

There are different scenarios that may occur during labor and birth that would require medical intervention. Most of them can be managed safely at home, while others will have better outcomes if they are treated at the hospital. A few rare, unpredictable emergencies may require immediate emergency transport to the hospital. The following are examples of emergencies which may occur during birth.

Cord Prolapse

Cord prolapse[162] occurs when the umbilical cord slips out of the uterus into the vagina prior to the birth of the baby. If the cord hangs out of the uterus, it can kink or be compressed. This may cause decreased blood flow to the baby, resulting in oxygen deprivation to the baby's brain and other vital organs.

How does it occur?

Cord prolapse can happen when the water breaks, either naturally or artificially, before the baby's head is fully engaged in the mother's pelvis. If the head is not blocking the cervix, the cord may slip down ahead of the baby.

Another risk factor for cord prolapse is at a breech birth, where the baby's feet come out ahead of the baby's head.

Delivery of twins or multiples has an increased risk[163] of cord prolapse, as Baby B's cord can slip out after Baby A is born.

Cord prolapse may also occur if the umbilical cord is unusually long.

What are the signs of cord prolapse?

The cord will be visible in the vagina. There may also be a drop in fetal heart rate.

Prolapsed cord is an indication for a c-section, and mom will need emergency transportation to the hospital.

Moms will be instructed to get into a knee-chest position, raising her bottom higher than her shoulders, and will remain in this position until she is in the operating room. If her midwife is with her, her midwife will put her fingers into the woman's vagina and lift the baby's head off the cord so that it is not compressed.

What are the chances of cord prolapse?

A prolapsed cord occurs in about 0.1% to 0.6%[164] of all births, although in recent years occurrence appears to be even lower than 0.1%.

Postpartum Hemorrhage (PPH)

You will continue to feel contractions after the placenta emerges as your uterus contracts and shrinks down to size. When the placenta detaches from the uterine wall, there are open blood vessels at the surface that are bleeding. It takes a few weeks for the area to heal and stop bleeding, and during that period of time the bleeding will lessen. Normally, a woman will lose up to 500 milliliters of blood during a vaginal delivery and up to 1000 millimeters in a c-section.

During pregnancy your blood volume increases by about 50%, so you can afford to lose some blood during birth without concern.

If the blood loss is more than 500 milliliters for a vaginal birth, and more than 1000 milliliters for a cesarean delivery, it is termed postpartum hemorrhage (PPH). PPH[165] occurs in about 3% of vaginal births and 5% of c-sections.

A woman having PPH will feel dizzy, light-headed, and nauseous. Her blood pressure will be low and her heart rate will be high.

The most common reason for PPH is uterine atony, which is when the uterus doesn't contract well after birth. Normally, if you massage your stomach after birth you should feel a hard ball. The tightening of your uterus helps close off the site where the placenta separated from the uterine wall. This prevents excessive bleeding. A sign of uterine atony is when the uterus feels soft and loose. If uterine atony is present, the midwife, doctor, or nurse will massage the uterus vigorously to stimulate it to contract.

Other causes of PPH include retained placenta, where pieces of the placenta are left inside. Your health care provider will inspect the placenta to ensure it is intact for this reason.

Another source for the excessive bleeding may be a cervical[166] or vaginal tear at the time of birth. Tears are more closely associated with an induction or assisted vaginal delivery. The tear will be repaired with stitches.

How is PPH treated?

PPH is treated at a home birth in the same way it is treated at the hospital:

1. The midwife massages the uterus, expelling any clots inside the uterus that are preventing the uterus from contracting.
2. Pitocin will be administered either via IV or via injection.
3. Mom will be asked to urinate. If she can't, a catheter will be inserted into her urethra to drain the bladder. This is because a full bladder may prevent the uterus from contracting effectively.

4. If the uterus is firm and the mom is still bleeding heavily, the midwife will inspect the vagina and cervix to determine if there are any large tears causing the bleeding. If any are found, they are repaired with stitches.

These steps usually stop a hemorrhage pretty quickly, and women with PPH usually recover well at home.

If the hemorrhage is severe, or if the bleeding restarts, an ambulance will be called for immediate transportation to the hospital.

Hemorrhages are less common at home births compared to hospital births. In 2012, a BMC Pregnancy & Childbirth research report[167] published in the United Kingdom reported that postpartum hemorrhage occurred more frequently at a planned hospital birth than at a planned home birth. Common interventions may be a factor causing postpartum hemorrhage. For example, there is a higher rate of postpartum hemorrhage with inductions[168] or labor augmentations when Pitocin is used. Doctors usually continue running Pitocin after the baby is born to keep the uterus contracting, preventing PPH. This mirrors the action that breastfeeding right after birth does. Breastfeeding stimulates oxytocin release, which causes uterine contractions and prevents PPH.

Chorioamnionitis

Chorioamnionitis is an infection of the membranes surrounding the baby and the amniotic fluid. It occurs in 2 to 4%[169] of births and commonly manifests as a mild infection requiring antibiotics. In rare cases, it can be more serious and the infection is transmitted to the baby. Once the water is broken, the sterile environment in the uterus is breached with the risk of infection remaining present until birth. For this reason, vaginal exams are minimized so as not to introduce infection in the uterus.

Nuchal Cord

Nuchal cord occurs when the umbilical cord is wrapped around the baby's neck. The umbilical cord subsists of Wharton's jelly, which is a gelatinous substance that coats and protects the arteries and vein inside it. This is the reason why nuchal cords do not usually cause any problems at birth.

If the cord is wrapped so tightly that it becomes compressed, oxygen rich blood may not reach the baby. In addition, if the cord compresses the carotid artery in the baby's neck, that will prevent blood supply from reaching the brain.

Another problematic scenario is if it wraps several times around the baby's neck or body, resulting in a shortened cord with less slack for the baby's descent. A c-section may be necessary if the baby has a difficult time descending.

A nuchal cord is present in 25% of pregnancies[170]. The vast majority of the time, the doctor or midwife will just slip the cord over the baby's head as the baby's head emerges.

Nuchal cord is primarily caused by normal fetal movements in utero. A very active baby will have a higher likelihood of nuchal cord. Other factors that will increase the odds of nuchal cord include being pregnant with multiples, having an unusually long umbilical cord, or having too much amniotic fluid (polyhydramnios).

How do you know if your baby has a nuchal cord before it's born?

The only way to tell is by having an ultrasound, but there is no medical indication to check before birth. The reason for that is because it is so unlikely for nuchal cord to be a problem. In addition, the baby's movements are unpredictable, and the cord may unwrap as baby flips back the other way.

If the baby's heart rate drops during labor, it may indicate a problem related to a nuchal cord. If a midwife spot checks the baby's heart rate during a contraction and finds a decel, where the baby's heart rate is dropping, this may be an indication to transport to the hospital for further observation and possible interventions.

Placental Abruption

Placental abruption occurs when the placenta partially or fully separates from the uterine wall. The baby receives its nourishment through its umbilical cord which is connected to the placenta that is attached to the uterine wall. Blood vessels run from the mom's blood vessels through the uterine wall to the placenta, bringing oxygen and nutrients the baby needs in order to grow and develop. If the placenta detaches from the wall of the uterus, the supply of oxygen and nutrients will be interrupted. How much this will impact mom and baby depends on how much of it separates. It can be a very slight separation with minimal bleeding or, very rarely, it could be a total separation. It may occur at some point during the third trimester, or it may occur during labor.

There are several risk factors for placental abruption which will increase a woman's chances of having one.

Suffering a fall or sustaining trauma to the abdomen can cause placental abruption. For example, a bad car accident or a fall down a flight of stairs.

Preeclampsia, or high blood pressure during pregnancy, may cause placental abruption, among other complications. A woman who develops preeclampsia during pregnancy will need to transfer care to an obstetrician.

Other risk factors[171] for placental abruption include smoking, alcohol use, and a previous c-section delivery[172].

According to a study[173] published in 2011, 0.4% to 1% of pregnancies have some degree of placental abruption occurring at any time during the third trimester.

If a slight placental abruption occurs during labor, the mother should be transported to the hospital for careful observation. A complete placental abruption will usually occur along with other risk factors which preclude a home birth. For example, a woman with preeclampsia would be under the care of an obstetrician.

Meconium Aspiration Syndrome (MAS)

Meconium is the first stool a newborn passes, usually within the first few hours after birth when they are having their first or second feeding.

Sometimes, a baby passes meconium while still in utero and then subsequently inhales it. If this happens, the baby may have difficulty breathing at birth.

Meconium is passed in utero in 10 to 15% of births, and 5 to 10%[174] of those babies will have some difficulty breathing at birth. If a baby is having difficulty breathing, they will need to be transported to the hospital for additional care and observation.

If a woman's water breaks and it is brown or green in color, this indicates meconium was passed by the baby. If that should happen, it is prudent to go to the hospital for the delivery, in case the baby has MAS at birth.

Another clue that meconium was passed would be a slowed fetal heart rate. A slowed heart rate indicates the baby is in distress, which may cause the baby to pass meconium. The mother may need to be transferred to the hospital if the baby is having decels.

According to a study[175] published in 2011, 82% of infants exposed to meconium-stained amniotic fluid at birth had an Apgar score above 7.

Amniotic fluid embolism (AFE)

Amniotic fluid embolism AFE[176] is an extremely rare occurrence where a bubble of amniotic fluid enters the mother's bloodstream. As it moves along in the blood stream it may lodge in the lungs, causing respiratory distress.

It statistically occurs in 2 per 100,000 deliveries[177] and is more likely to occur during an induction or just after a c-section.

Hospitalization is needed for treatment, although mortality rates are high even with immediate intervention in a hospital. This is because AFE often leads to disseminated intravascular coagulation (DIC).

Disseminated Intravascular Coagulation (DIC)

Occurring in around 3 per 10,000 births[178], DIC is a bleeding disorder that requires immediate transportation to the hospital for treatment.

It is a rare complication which may be caused by a retained placenta, placental abruption, preeclampsia, amniotic fluid embolism, or postpartum hemorrhage, among other disorders.

The mortality rate for mothers who have DIC is 6.25%.

I know the medical complications discussed in this chapter are worrisome, but it is important to know and understand the risks involved when planning a home birth. Keep in mind though, a well-trained midwife will not only be able to handle common complications but more importantly, will know when to transfer mom to the hospital before it becomes an emergency.

CHAPTER 9
The Dutch Maternity System

The World Bank Data[179] released the Maternal Mortality Ratio in 2019. It provides statistics on maternal deaths per 100,000 births from the years 2000-2017. According to this data, the United States' maternal mortality rate is 19 per 100,000 births. The United Kingdom's maternal mortality rate is 7 maternal deaths per 100,000 births. The Netherlands' (Holland's) maternal mortality rate is 5 maternal deaths per 100,000 births.

The United States has one of the highest rates of doctors delivering babies in the world. Holland and Great Britain, on the other hand, are countries where every pregnant woman sees a midwife, as long as she has no preexisting medical conditions and no complications during her pregnancy and birth. Based on this data, you can infer that low-risk women have better outcomes seeing a midwife than seeing an obstetrician.

Renske Kuiper[180], a midwife living and practicing in Holland, explains the structure of the Dutch maternity system:

> In Holland we have a VIL. We call a midwife Verloskundige in Dutch, so VIL stands for Verloskundige Indication List. It is a system where an A, B, C, and D indication is assigned to a woman when she enters the maternity system.
>
> A is assigned for midwifery care/primary care.
>
> C is for obstetrician/gynecologists and secondary care (there are also midwives working in hospitals).
>
> B is an indication where the woman is at lower risk than C indication, and where the midwife collaborates with an obstetrician.
>
> D is a place indication for hospital birth (but can be with your primary care midwife).
>
> When a woman goes into labor, they call us, and if the woman is low-risk, we go to their house to see if they are in labor and how they are doing. After we examine them, the woman can still decide where they want to deliver. We are able to deliver the baby at home or in the hospital. In both cases, whether it's at home or in the hospital, if we think there might be a problem, we will refer to the obstetrician. If they are at home they will be transported to the hospital if needed.

Carina Primavesi[181], an Italian-Brazilian mom, had her first home birth in Holland with Renske Kuiper. Carina initially shared the following home birth story on her personal Facebook account. She hoped to inspire women with her birth story and to show people what an empowering experience birth can be. Carina's story contrasts the care she experienced with her first pregnancy when she lived in Italy where she gave birth with a doctor in the hospital, with her second child's home birth in Holland with a midwife. Carina gave me permission to share her story in this book.

Carina's Story

I started to practice pregnancy yoga with Maria Laura, a wonderful teacher, in Milan in 2015. She planted a seed in my mind, as she would say, "Birth is much easier outside the hospital, in a birthing center (or at home), without medical interventions. There you can relax, and the delivery goes so much smoother, quicker and with less pain." So, I started to read more about it, talked with some friends, and I was convinced that I wanted to have my baby in a more natural way: in a birth center, in the bath, with a doula.

However, my husband did not like the idea as he thought that the birth would be safer in a hospital. Since it was my first delivery and I did not know exactly what to expect, I didn't insist and gave up on this idea. I instead chose to go to the hospital for my delivery. I decided to prepare my body (yoga, special positions, breathings) to have at least a natural delivery without any pain killers, despite being in the hospital.

When I was at 40 weeks, I went to an appointment in the hospital, and they told me I did not have enough amniotic fluid (later, I realized that it was not true, since I was feeling my daughter moving a lot like always). They wanted to induce my labour with oxytocin at that moment! I was terrified! I told them I was feeling my daughter moving a lot, and they decided to attach the electronic fetal monitor on my belly. They noticed that she was moving well, but I still needed to sign that it was my responsibility to not let them induce me. However, I allowed them to rupture my membranes (since they convinced me it was the safest solution in my case). At 3:30 a.m. the next day, my labour started. It was a very painful and traumatic labour of fourteen hours. I gave up my idea of having an all-natural delivery and decided to have an epidural in the hospital. The anesthesiologist came very late though, and the pushing phase was very long and tough. It was exhausting. At least my baby was born with a good Apgar score, the most important thing in the end.

It was very far away from the delivery I was dreaming of having. I came back home telling everybody that my newborn baby would be my only child! The postpartum period was very hard as well.

To clarify, I would like to highlight that my first birth was, as it was, not because it happened in Italy, but because of the circumstances surrounding it. I could have been in any other country and would have had the same result.

After six months, we moved to Amsterdam, and by the end of the year I got pregnant with my second. And here the nice story starts... Instead of an obstetrician, a midwife was making my monthly checks only by checking my belly, my baby's heartbeat, and my blood pressure. I had 3 ultrasounds during the whole pregnancy (instead of the 8 I had during my first pregnancy). I had only 1 blood test (instead of 8 during my first pregnancy). The midwives were always so kind and warm with me that I began to feel secure, even though I never went to the hospital (even after birth). The most surprising part for me was when I had any cramps, pain, headache, nausea or anything disturbing me, my midwife team told me just to listen to my body and do what it was asking for (relax, sleep more, sit, do not walk much) with no medicine prescribed at all. Meanwhile, during my first pregnancy, the doctors were always prescribing me medication for every kind of pain or symptom (which I never took since I do not like to take medication if it is not strictly necessary).

Looking for a prenatal course, I found a wonderful hypnobirthing course. It taught you a new vocabulary to use to describe labor and birth, breaking the traditional association of birth with pain. It teaches that when a woman feels fear during childbirth, her body releases stress hormones that trigger the body's "fight or flight" response. This causes muscles to tighten and increases the duration and pain of the birthing process. By training the subconscious mind through meditation, breathing, affirmations, and visualizations, it teaches you how to have a safe, gentle and smoother birth. It can happen at home, at a birthing center, or in the hospital, wherever you feel safer.

I practiced at least one of their techniques almost every day in the last 2 months of my pregnancy. I tried my best to avoid the experience that I had with my first delivery. This time, I trained my body (through yoga and exercise) and my mind, which I didn't do in the first pregnancy, but it was the most important factor, in my opinion, to having a smoother birth.

The wish to give birth in the bath, without any painkillers, was coming back. Since a lot of women give birth at home here, I mentioned this idea to my husband again. He continued to say that he would prefer a hospital birth. Fortunately, I found the best solution: a birthing center, a place with rooms equipped with baths, beautifully decorated, and endowed with every comfort to deliver the baby, in a safe homey place. This one was connected to a hospital, where I could have gone to if any problem happened or if I wished for a painkiller at the last minute. So, we were both satisfied!

When I was 40 weeks, I had my check-up with the midwife at her office (Het Geboortecentrum Amsterdam). She only asked me if I still was feeling the baby moving like always (not less than normal), how I was feeling, and if I had any doubts about my delivery. She touched my belly to check if the baby was in an optimal position, checked the baby's heart rate, and checked my blood pressure. There was no ultrasound or electronic fetal monitoring. She told me to observe the movements of my baby (they should not decrease), to trust in my body that it knows the right time to give birth, and go back home to relax, while I still have time.

One week later, there was no sign that my daughter wanted to come out. I had the 41 weeks check-up. The midwife did the same procedures as the last time, and also suggested that she sweep the membranes when I would be 41 weeks + 3 days. If that didn't work, she would do another membrane sweep at 41 weeks + 5 days. If that still didn't work, 2 days later, I would become a "medical pregnancy" at 42 weeks. That meant I would be directed to an obstetrician, and I would to decide which doctor and hospital (not the birthing center anymore) I would give birth at. I needed to decide what I preferred to do if my daughter was not born by the time I was 42 weeks— artificial oxytocin, etc.

When I was 41 weeks + 3 days, I had no signs of labor at all. A lot of friends and relatives were asking me how I could be that far advanced in my pregnancy without having further check-ups. They said the baby may not be doing well in my belly, the baby may grow larger than my body could support, and my placenta may be too aged to feed my baby, etc… So, I called Inbal, my teacher from Isis Hypnobirthing & Yoga, to ask her what I could do to stimulate my daughter to come out. She answered by asking me, "Are you feeling well? Is your baby growing well?"

I answered positive for both questions. "So, if you have no medical reason to rush things forward, you could ask your midwife for alternatives besides sweeping the membranes and discuss what else can be done. Plus, practicing some of the hypnobirthing tools will help you be in a more relaxed and calm state, the best way to set the ground for a natural onset of birth." After this call, I decided to wait one more day and increase the meditation time.

The day after, 41 weeks + 4 days, I confess, I was very anxious. I booked an hour and thirty minutes of reflexology with Hilde from De Voetnoodt, to help unblock any emotion and whatever was necessary to have a better labor. It was the best decision of the day! I came back home full of energy and feeling very relaxed, with more patience and trust while I waited to meet my baby.

The next day, I started to have some mild contractions. My husband stayed home as we thought the day had arrived! But the contractions lasted all day long without any further progress. I called the midwife to tell her and she told me that it could also mean nothing. And she agreed to come over the next morning to my home to do a check-up and rupture my membranes (break my water) if I did not want to be transferred to an obstetrician, meaning, in case my daughter did not arrive before 42 weeks, the birth would have been in the hospital, not in the birthing center. The membrane sweep would be my last chance to have my dream birth in the bath. However, to me, it also meant I wouldn't have a natural birth, since rupturing the membranes does not respect the natural timing of a baby's birth; it begins the process of birth for a baby who is not yet ready to be born. I had many doubts which way would be better:

respect my baby's time or try to have my water birth in a natural way before 42 weeks.

That evening, I meditated and tried to relax, visualizing my water birth and listening to soft music with lit candles. During the last few months of my pregnancy, I was feeling a little afraid to have a water birth without any pain killers. However, after waiting so long (every day after 40 weeks seemed never ending), I was dreaming about this moment without fear.

Around 3:00-3:10 a.m., I woke up with stronger contractions. I was still not very convinced that this was it. They were bearable, so I went into the living room to exercise on my yoga ball. My husband woke up with me, and I told him to go back to sleep since it could still take a long time (it is said the second labour could last half the first, so I was expecting around 7 hours). I counted the first contractions, and they were still irregular. Around 3:30 a.m., they became more frequent and stronger, so I decided to wait at least 30 minutes to see if they were really regular. My husband was worried and came to see if I was okay. I told him again to go back to sleep as I thought it was just the beginning of the process as they were still not painful. After 15 minutes they started to become a little bit painful, so my husband wanted to call the midwife. Here in Holland, you do not go to the hospital alone; you need to call your midwife to check you first at home and then you go together with her to the selected hospital or birthing center. I would have waited longer since those contractions were similar to my first daughter's early labor. After his insistence (fortunately!), we called the midwife at 3:51 a.m., and she came around 20 minutes later.

When she arrived, she checked me and said, "You are already too far, we will stay at home!"

I said, "What???" I couldn't believe that!

She said again, "You are almost fully dilated. We do not have time to go to the hospital."

My husband, my mother (who was here for the birth), and I were quite shocked! It was my initial plan to give birth at home, but to be honest, I hadn't really prepared myself for that. So, it was a very unexpected surprise! Of course I was happy that I could realize my original dream. Since I trusted in myself and in my body, the contractions kept up and became even stronger, but not more painful. During the entire labor, I was practicing hypnobirthing techniques.

We took our krampakket, a box that the insurance sends when you are pregnant in Holland, with everything you need in case you want/need to give birth at home. The midwife asked my husband for a few things: towels, clothes, things for the baby (which were all in my hospital bag) and other things that I could not pay attention to. She went back to her car to get her emergency equipment. I asked my husband to fill the bath with water.

After 25 minutes, my midwife arrived, my water broke, and I suddenly started to feel very strong pressure from the baby! The midwife told me to go into the bath which was finally full.

After a few rounds of breathing and 3 contractions, which occurred within about 5 minutes, my daughter came out! At 4:50 a.m., with an explosion of emotions, I could only cry from happiness as I held my baby in my arms, thinking how incredible nature is! My body could make it! Alone, without any medical intervention, without any painkillers, only me and my mind! And the best thing: I could erase my past birth experience, which was full of pain, and replace it with a beautiful, minimally painful, soothing home birth experience.

It was not my relaxed and quiet water birth with just some music and candles that I had dreamed of. But somehow, it was much better! My body worked well to deliver my daughter quickly and smoothly. Everything was perfect. The baby was born weighing 4 kilograms (8.8 pounds). I didn't have any difficulty because of it since I learned from hypnobirthing that my baby's size is perfect to my body (but I'm still glad I didn't know her weight before the birth!).

It was one of the most wonderful experiences I have had in my life: feeling the power of my body, going beyond the birth beliefs of my culture (the Brazilian side full of C-sections and the Italian side with inductions and painkillers), trusting in my body and fulfilling a dream. A few friends said that my subconscious had planned on giving birth at home without telling anybody (who knows?).

I also would like to highlight that this postpartum period was much easier for me. My second baby is much calmer and more easy-going than my older baby. First of all, because I waited for her to come naturally, without forcing her out with any kind of induction, her body was ready and able to adapt to our world. Secondly, my daughter was given to me for skin-to-skin contact for the first two hours after birth without any check-ups (the vitamin k shot and the other exams were done after a few days), creating a stronger and important first bonding. Third, I had a Kraamzorg² for eight days after birth at home to check my baby and me, to help with breastfeeding, and whatever was necessary, including housework. We didn't need to leave home for any reason during these days. This let me relax more and I could start our life in a smoother, more restful way.

I never thought I'd say this one day, but I would like to go back to that day just to feel all the emotions again, to feel my body experiencing this home birth in the perfect way that it should be for every woman. This is how it was for our grandmothers.

───────────

2   *Kraamzorg – The maternity care in Holland is totally unique. No other country in the world has this kind of maternity care where a professional maternity nurse looks after a mother and her new born baby during the first few days after birth. A Kraamzorg's primary responsibility is to ensure that the mother's recovery is quick and efficient and that the baby's development is evolving appropriately. The nurse will show you how to care for your new born baby, for example, how to breastfeed properly. She will look after older children and make sure that meals are prepared, take care of laundry and light household cleaning. If you have visitors, she will help arrange a time that doesn't interrupt with your baby's and your rest. If you have a home birth, she will also be there after the birth to clean up.*

Unfortunately, nowadays, birth is so medicalized. Our culture is full of beliefs that we need doctors, hospital, inductions, as well as a lot of exams and checks in order to give birth, the most natural thing in the world! Of course, there are cases where the mother really does need some help and support from the doctors (which is very appreciated). But some of them (in Brazil, most of them) are done without any reason. After having my second child here in Holland, I have realized my dream and I am very glad to be here!

Carina's beautiful home birth story highlights the Dutch maternity care system, which is very supportive of women throughout pregnancy, childbirth, and beyond. The Dutch attitude toward pregnancy is that pregnancy is not an illness and, therefore, a doctor is unwarranted unless a medical need is present.

When do women in Holland need to decide if they would like to have a home birth? Dr. Ank de Jonge, Dutch midwife and researcher, explains in an interview[182]:

> In Holland, you don't have to choose before your birth. I have to ask what you intend to do, but you can easily change your mind, because everyone starts birth at home. You can see how you feel, and if you feel like, "I'm not going anywhere, let's stay here," that's fine. We've got stuff with us, and the initial stages are exactly the same wherever you want to give birth. So that means if you suddenly go too fast or you don't want to move, you can just give birth. If you wanted to give birth at home and you decide you want medication, or you don't like it (at home), then you can still go to hospital. The system gives you a lot of flexibility.
>
> The system in Holland is very strong. That part of the system in Holland is very strong. I even talked to an obstetrician last week who said the same: women should stay at home as long as they can because we know from

all the literature it is better for them. And of course, even if they want to have the actual birth in hospital, it's so great that someone can be at your home during the initial stages. It's very stressful to know when you should move to hospital, especially if you've had a quick birth before. Women get very nervous. Here, you don't have to be. You call the midwife and she'll be at your place, which is great. Quite frequently, especially with second or more babies, women plan to give birth in hospital but then end up at home, and then they are happy because that means it usually went very smoothly.

One time, I remember that I had a birth with a lady from Morocco or Turkey, and usually ethnic minority women are more likely to want to give birth in hospital, because they come from countries where home birth is not that safe, and they feel that they're now they are in a rich country and they want the benefits of a hospital. One lady was too quick, and she gave birth at home. The husband was so surprised when he saw me bringing in all the stuff we carry, and he said, "Oh, but you've got everything with you, then we might as well stay at home," which made me realize we should inform women more about all the equipment that we bring.

We carry oxygen, we carry all the tools for the birth, we can do an episiotomy, we can suture. People sometimes don't realize that we've got all the things with us. There's sometimes so much misunderstanding, they think we only come with a screwdriver or something.

CHAPTER 10

What Does the Research Say About Home Birth?

A s of 2015, Holland has the highest home birth rate in the developed world at 13%.[183] In comparison, other countries' home birth rates are 0.6% in Finland, 0.9% in the United States, 3.3% in New Zealand, 0.3% in Australia, 1.4% in Canada, and 2.3% in England.

In 2010, the BMJ[184] published a study comparing perinatal outcomes among European countries. Holland's perinatal outcomes rated poorly compared to other European countries. Because home birth is such an integral part of the Dutch maternity system, it was blamed as the cause for the poor neonatal outcomes.

Professor Tamar van Haaren-ten Haken[185], Dutch midwife and author of The Place to Be[186], discusses the home birth studies in an interview I had with her.

Well, the first numbers were from 2004. It was the first time that results were published comparing European data. This data showed that the Netherlands was not doing well on perinatal mortality. Everyone was pointing to our system because what was different between the Netherlands and other countries is we have a lot of home births. So what was happening was that before we really looked at what's going on and what the numbers were telling us, everybody was already pointing at our home birth system. So we did the research again (re-analysis) in 2008 and there was a new report with the same data, so we looked more in detail at what was happening here, and we saw that it was very difficult to compare all European countries because of the difference in registration level. We have quite a good registration level in the Netherlands, but for all other countries: when are you registering a perinatal mortality? From how many weeks till how many weeks after birth? So there was quite a lot of difference when registering the data. We also saw differences between the populations.

The mean age for when women have their first baby is quite high in the Netherlands compared to other countries, but that doesn't really explain all the numbers. The Netherlands had a different approach to premature birth. In Germany, for instance, they are actively taking care for babies that are born from 24 weeks gestation, whereas in the Netherlands, we have a more conservative approach in case of a very premature neonate. There are so many problems with morbidity and neurologic development with very premature babies, so that was also a difference between European countries, because are you keeping babies alive with high morbidity rates later on or choosing not to give treatment for very premature babies? So I think it's a combination of culture, a combination of population, and a combination of how we are registering all the data. What is very interesting about the study is we were not the highest rate of perinatal mortality. The highest number was in France. And France is a country where birth is highly medicalized. Everyone gives birth in hospitals there, so I think it's very complex.

On the other hand, I think it was a good moment to reflect on our maternity care system. Until that moment, we always said, "Oh, we're doing so well in the Netherlands with a high home birth rate and very good numbers." Now we are thinking, "Is that really the point?" So what is happening since 2008 is that there are a lot of changes in maternity care in the Netherlands. We are going to more integrated care, more collaboration with all the different care providers, but also with the goal to preserve the different choices of place for birth. We are not outlawing home birth, as far as I know, although I can't see in the future.

We had some problems with those studies but I think it is also a good point that you can be critical and reflect on your own maternity care system. The latest European data from 2015 shows that the neonatal mortality rate in the Netherlands has gone down. Recent studies also show no connection between infant mortality and home births.

This 2015 research study[187] was done by Dr. Ank de Jonge[188] comparing women with low-risk pregnancies and their perinatal outcomes at hospital births, to the same population at planned home births. The study showed no difference between the two settings, and it exonerates the home birth system in Holland. Unfortunately, much damage was already done in the public's perception of home birth safety, and Holland's home birth rate is in decline.

Ank spoke about it with me in an interview:

> We've had a lot of bad press over the last decade or so, so that hasn't helped; it has decreased confidence among people in home birth. I'm still practicing as a midwife, and I find I have people who I would call typical "home birthers" now questioning whether it's safe, and if the women feel it's safe, then the family doesn't think so. So we have the same lack of confidence other countries have had for a long time.

Holland is unique in that the system is set up to support home birth safely. Ank observes:

> In case of an emergency, the ambulance knows what to do. Women get to hospital in time, and I think people forget that. If you look at other countries, if you read between the lines, about 1 in 200 or so babies are born before arrival, so that's quite a number.
>
> Women in England and other countries give birth in the car park, or in a taxi, or wherever, whereas in Holland, if a woman gives birth fast, a midwife can be with her usually in time, or at least in time for the placenta, and have all of her equipment with her. So that's an added benefit of having a home birth system. Women always start at home in Holland, so if someone goes into labor, even if they want to give birth in hospital, they always call the midwife. The midwife then comes to the house, assesses the situation, and then if they're not in labor, they have a cup of tea and the midwife reassures them, makes a plan with them, and discusses when she'll come back.

This is in contrast to having a hospital birth in another country: you go to the hospital, you're sent home because you're too early, you go back again, then you're sent home again. You don't have that in Holland. Midwives will come to your house as often as needed and then go with you to the hospital if you want to give birth there and continue your care there. So it's not only about giving birth at home. It's a whole system where you can be at home as long as you're comfortable at home, so even if you want to give birth in hospital, you can be at home and then go to hospital when labor is progressing, or you can change your mind.

In the UK[189], Britain's national health service recommends healthy women with low-risk pregnancies deliver their babies at home or at birthing centers. The support came after Great Britain ran a landmark study on home birth, called the Birthplace Study[190]. They researched 64,538 women with low-risk pregnancies giving birth at home, at freestanding birth centers, and at hospitals between April 2008 and April 2010. When the results came in, they found no difference in risk between hospital births and home births for women who have previously given birth.

A significant finding that came up though, is that there were slightly poorer outcomes associated with home births for women having their first baby. For first-time mothers, adverse perinatal outcome events were 9.3 per 1000 births for planned home births, compared with 5.3 per 1000 births for planned hospital births. There was also a higher hospital transfer rate for first-time mothers at a rate of 36 to 45%, compared to 9 to 13% for women who had previously given birth.

Another birthplace study[191] worth looking at was done in Canada. It studied outcomes of hospital births and home births taking place between January 2000 through December 2004 in British Columbia. Results showed the rate of perinatal death at a home birth per 1000 births was 0.35, a hospital birth attended by a midwife was 0.57, and a hospital birth attended by a physician was 0.64.

In 2015, a new Canadian birthplace study[192] was published comparing outcomes of home births and outcomes of hospital births. Researcher Dr. Eileen Hutton and her team looked through data on 23,000 births in Canada over a three-year period between 2006 and 2009. They compared outcomes for mothers who planned a home birth with mothers who planned a hospital birth. The study showed home births were just as safe as hospital births for low-risk moms, when home birth takes place in a health care system where home birth is well integrated. Canadian midwives are rigorously trained and have a rigid system where they cannot deliver a baby at home unless specific criteria are met.

Holland, Great Britain, and Canada are all countries where home birth is well supported both on a medical and societal level. There are studies done in other countries where outcomes were not as good.

Dr. Ank de Jonge[193] points out,

> We have published a lot on home birth. We did the largest studies[194] on home birth because we have the most home births in the Western world, and I find we don't see any difference in perinatal outcomes, and better maternal outcomes even, for planned home births compared to planned hospital birth. Sometimes people take that and say, "Oh, see, home birth is safe" and then apply it to other systems. We are always careful in our conclusions to say that what we find is in a context of well-trained midwives, a good referral system, and a competent transportation system, and in that context, we see good outcomes. I think

you have to be careful when translating it to systems where either people are not well trained, or you have a problem with transport, or your hospital is completely hostile to home birth. In these situations you may have different outcomes. You see that actually in the U.S. You have a study from Oregon showing poor birth outcomes for planned home births or planned birth center births, which included all out-of-hospital births. The poor outcomes may be attributed to lay midwives and unsupervised home births. When you don't have good guidelines, then the outcomes may not be as good.

The Oregon home birth study[195], which was published in 2015 in the *New England Journal of Medicine,* showed that in the state of Oregon, home births have worse outcomes than hospital births. This study drew data from Oregon state birth certificates from the years 2012 and 2013. They found that the incidence of infant deaths at home births were 3.9 per 1000 births, compared to 1.8 per 1000 births at hospitals.

The *Midwifery Today*[196] journal explains that the reason neonatal death rate was higher at home births in this 2015 study is because the researchers lumped all out-of-hospital births together, including unplanned and unassisted home births.

Other critics[197] point out that the locale where the study took place has little regulation over midwives to ensure they are up to par with current midwifery standards. Some of the midwives[198] have little formal training and may be inexperienced with birth emergencies. They may not recognize signs of fetal distress, or they may choose to continue to care for women who have pregnancy complications, such as preeclampsia.

Ank explains further:

> There's a lot of variation in the US, with different levels of
> midwives and no consistent quality, so that makes it more
> difficult to interpret. I'm saying this because in Holland,
> we are always close to a hospital. We've got a system that's
> prepared for home birth. It's a very different thing when
> you're in the US somewhere, hours away from a hospital
> that's hostile to even receive you. I think that is the reason
> why you have to sometimes be careful when interpreting
> research study findings.
>
> When the Oregon study came out, I was invited to an
> online panel from the *New England Journal of Medicine*,
> where it was published. It was actually very interesting.
> We had an online discussion with obstetricians from the
> US and they were saying that they looked at countries like
> UK and Holland and they said, "Look, we can see in these
> countries that it can be safe to plan your birth at home.
> We know in the US, even though we tell women that they
> should give birth in hospital, some of them don't, so why
> don't we stop pressuring them and just set up a system
> that's safe for them to choose home birth if they want to.
> So at least treat them with respect when they are referred,
> as well as make sure there are guidelines for home birth."
> And I think that's a very good development. There's a lot
> to be done.

Midwifery in the United States is not standardized like it is in
Canada or Holland. Whereas in other countries a midwife requires
a college education in order to practice, in the United States many
home birth midwives are lay midwives, and do not hold a degree.

April Davis[199], an EMT and doula living in Utah, describes her background and experience with home birth:

> When I did emergency medical training as an 18-year-old, I was told if you have a home birth, you are absolutely crazy and everyone dies.
>
> Because EMTs really only see the crashes.
>
> They just see the worst-case scenarios for home births, and much of the time it's accidental home births or irresponsible midwives.
>
> Midwifery is not well-regulated here in Utah, and a lot of women do not understand that, so they'll hire one of these midwives who often have little to no training and just don't have the experience that they should have if they're going to be out on their own delivering babies.
>
> So my initial training that home birth is a terrible idea makes complete sense, but the more I looked into it, the more I started to realize that home births, especially when attended by a certified nurse midwife (CNM), typically have better outcomes than even hospital births.
>
> It's just so hard to look at statistics if they're not actually separated out whether the home birth was intended and who was attending!

Many medical personnel in some parts of the world have preconceived notions about women who plan a home birth and of the home birth midwives who support it. This lack of understanding and possible hostility to women who transfer to the hospital from a planned home birth may lead to suboptimal care and a negative birth experience for moms. In addition, a poor reception at a hospital transfer may lead the midwife to think twice before transferring another home birth patient to the hospital.

They may choose to wait too long to transfer a subsequent patient to the hospital, leading to poor outcomes. This is an example of why it is so beneficial to have a maternity system where home birth is supported and integrated.

Dr. Eugene (Gene) Declercq is a professor of community health sciences at Boston University and developer of the website Birth By Numbers.[200] In an interview[201] with me regarding how to read the research on the safety of home birth he reveals, "The biggest studies thus far were the ones out of the Netherlands that looked at it from the perspective of perinatal mortality and later neonatal mortality, and they found no differences in outcomes between low-risk hospital and home births. The other major study was the birthplace study in England, which also found no overall difference, but a higher risk for primipara mothers (first-time mothers). These all assume a low-risk population that they're screening beforehand."

As far as Gene's personal take on home birth, he discloses, "I support home birth for low-risk mothers working with well-trained midwives and where there is a whole structure around it and a backup system. Referral to a hospital shouldn't be something that's done in opposition to everything the hospital believes in, which is why in England women register for their home births at a hospital."

"Home and Birth Center Birth in the United States" is a study[202] published in May 2019 by Aaron Coughey and Melissa Cheyney. This study reviews the statistical findings of previous studies on the safety of birth centers and home births in the United States. The authors analyze the Netherlands and United Kingdom models of midwifery care and home birth and how they are integrated into the maternity system. They conclude that model collaboration between home birth midwives and obstetricians is critical to improving the safety of home birth in the United States, and bringing it up to par with other wealthy countries.

Gene states, "In judging the research, one of the things about the May 2019 study was they use an external standard for what a quality study is, instead of bringing personal biases to their assessment of the existing research, which at least gives you something to base your judgment on.

The other piece that's important is that Melissa Cheyney is a home birth midwife and anthropologist, and she does magnificent research in this area. But equally important, the other author, Aaron Caughey, is one of the most respected obstetrician researchers in the country, and what makes it an important piece is that it's jointly written by them."

When Gene was asked what conclusion that piece reached, he responds, "In the right supported circumstances, home birth is a viable option."

CHAPTER 11

How to Plan a Safe Home Birth

What a safe home birth looks like can differ between people and communities. For example, some women choose to have their babies unassisted at home, in a trend known as free birthing. They are basically delivering their baby on their own without a health care provider present.

Hannah Dahlen[203], an Australian midwife and professor of midwifery, wrote a book, *The Canary in the Coal Mine*[204], that discusses this trend and links it to a failure in maternity health care systems.

Hannah addresses this trend in an interview[205]:

> ...there are more people now probably free birthing at home without anyone in attendance, or no registered midwife in attendance, than there are home births with registered midwives.
>
> If you look at the whole of Australia and how many midwives are providing private home birth services, there are about 240 midwives. That's a very small number for the entire nation, and they're dropping every year because of

this reporting and victimization that is happening. So we know there are more women who free birth, who choose to birth without a midwife, now than there are births with a midwife. This happens because they either can't find a midwife, they can't afford them, or they're too far away. They live in rural, remote areas where there are no private midwives. They may also be so traumatized by the system and their experience with health providers that they don't even trust midwives.

The US has got the same situation of rising rates of free birth, hence why we're writing this book, *The Canary in the Coal Mine*. We're not listening to the women who are telling us the system is traumatizing them. There are not enough options. They're seeking midwifery care. They're seeking relationship-based care. We're continuing to ignore it, so they go off and they do their own thing. Then we turn around and we demonize them when it's actually our fault for not meeting women's needs.

While women have different reasons for choosing a free birth, it's important to acknowledge that many women have limited options. Maybe they live out in a rural community,[206] where the local hospital has a high c-section rate and routinely separates babies from their mothers for several hours after birth for observation. Some women may only have a local midwife who never went through the process to become legal. Everyone's circumstances are different.

Hannah Dahlen[207] states so eloquently in our interview:

We think only good mothers are mothers who sacrifice their needs for their baby. That's society's belief. However, good mothers are strong mothers, they're competent mothers, they're empowered mothers, and we're not getting that with the way we are risking childbirth to the point where we're devastating the hand that rocks the cradle. And we then sit there and wonder why we're ending up with the dysfunctions that we're seeing in children. We're not valuing women enough. If we valued women, really valued women, we'd get it right.

Mothers fare better at planned home births, as evidenced by a 2018 study[208]. It compared outcomes of low-risk pregnancies in high income countries according to their place of birth. They found that women planning home births have much lower rates of medical intervention. They also have significantly lower odds of a NICU admission. Across the board, home birth midwives have much lower c-section rates than hospital midwives and doctors. Some women will plan a home birth in order to lower their chance of have a c-section.

When it comes down to managing the risks at a planned home birth, the American College of Obstetricians and Gynecologists[209] discusses several factors that can make a difference. The first is hiring a home birth midwife who's accreditation meets the standards set by the International Confederation of Midwives Global Standards for Midwifery Education[210].

Choosing a competent midwife is critical. Selena tells a heart wrenching story of fetal loss because of her midwife's incompetence:

> It was a lay midwife who was seeing me, and this was my sixth pregnancy. I was 31 weeks and 2 days and she was ignoring my high blood pressure, telling me that it was psychological, that there's something I'm not talking about. I was like, "I had five other children normally."

She said, "What are you not telling me? There's something you're not telling me." She felt my high blood pressure was somehow related to my psychological state.

I had a placental abruption, caused by the high blood pressure, and I was bleeding. I went into the hospital and they found the baby had died. They had to induce me, and it was the only hospital birth I ever had.

I was walking around with really high blood pressure, and she should have sent me for medical attention. As a midwife, I would never allow someone to walk around with high blood pressure. I would send them to the doctor or the hospital and certainly not plan a home birth for them. This midwife had lost other babies as well. She had done 2 VBACs at home, and the babies had died. She is not practicing anymore.

It is so important to practice safe home birth and maintain a safe standard: single baby, head down, no blood pressure issues, and no other medical problems.

Selena went on to become a CNM, and strives to provide a safe home birth experience for her clients.

Selena's story has a number of lessons, primarily the importance of choosing a competent midwife who is well-trained and follows appropriate safety measures, including the transfer of care to an obstetrician for any medical conditions that arise during pregnancy.

In 2018, Dr. Eugene DeClerq published a paper[211] where he lists what criteria should be present for a safe home birth. It includes the following:

- A single baby, head down, at full term gestation
- Mom has no preexisting serious medical or obstetrical conditions and an absence of contraindications to a vaginal birth.

- The prenatal care, labor, birth, and postpartum care are attended by a licensed birth professional.
- Good communication and mutual respect between home birth providers and hospital staff when a woman is transferred from home to hospital.

An example of guidelines put out by a government to provide a safe home birth experience is the clinical directive,[212] published in 2018 by South Australia. It has very specific guidelines surrounding planned home birth, and you can read an excerpt as follows:

> The woman planning to give birth at home should be cared for by two registered midwives (one of whom is accredited to attend a planned home birth). They must:

- Ensure at least one of the registered midwives is in attendance at all times from the commencement of active labour until at least four hours post-birth of the baby.
- Ensure two registered midwives (one of whom is accredited to attend a planned home birth), are in attendance at all times from the commencement of the second stage of labour up until the completion of the third stage of labour.

To be accredited as competent in planned home birth, the registered midwife must:
- Have participated in at least five planned home births under supervision
- Practice according to the Planned Birth at Home in SA 2018 Clinical Directive
- Be aware of potential situational challenges that may arise during birth at home
- Have competency in maternal and neonatal resuscitation, intravenous cannulation, perineal suturing, and newborn examination (as directed by local Policies).

Other items included are that the pregnancy must be between 37 and 42 weeks gestation and only involve a single baby head down. The home birth must take place at a home that is within 30 minutes traveling time by ambulance from the participating hospital. The home must have reliable phone coverage, clean running water, electricity, and be clean and hygienic.

Home birth doula Ruthie Pearlman[213] tells us how she responds to women who are worried about birth emergencies occurring at a planned home birth:

> I explain that the midwives are trained and know how to handle these situations. They come with oxygen. They come with Pitocin. They know what to do. They know infant CPR. They will massage a bleeding uterus for as long as it takes until they get to the hospital and are able to take their hands away.
>
> If you consider they're at the same level as doctors and nurses in the hospital, and know what to do, you have all the benefit of being in your home in your own space without exposing yourself and your baby to the foreign germs. And without all the interruptions that happen in the hospital, a home birth is a good, safe choice.

Barbara Ben Ami[214], Israeli home birth midwife, shares her story:

> My personal story is I went to nursing school and became a midwife. I was vehemently anti-home birth. I thought home birth was dangerous, reckless, and negligent, and completely insane. How could you endanger your baby because you wanted a certain experience!?! That's exactly what I thought. And to all of my friends who talked to me about home birth, I told them, "No, I'll give you a home birth in the hospital." That's where I came from; I am a very medical person.

I met up with homeopathy because I went to a family physician with one of my kids, and she gave them homeopathic treatment that worked like magic, and I thought, "Oh my gosh, what was that? I have to check that out." Then I did a course for midwives called Natural Childbirth, and I had a few home birth midwives who came to speak with us. There were only three then in the whole country. I talked to one of them during the break and I said, "It sounds really nice what you're telling me, but you know as well as I do that catastrophes can happen at birth, and birth can change in a second, and how can you be so irresponsible?"

And I remember she looked at me and said, "Why don't you just come along with me to a home birth and check it out?" Suddenly something happened to me and I said, "You know what? Okay."

I came with her to a home birth, and it completely changed my life. We worked together. It was a very long, difficult first birth. She pushed out a huge baby, trying out all these different positions. I know how it would have ended in the hospital. It was amazing, and I remember walking out. My husband drove me there because there was no GPS. This was 20 years ago. I woke him up, as he was sleeping in the car, and I said to him, "Oh my God, I've made a mistake. I've been doing the wrong thing for all these years." I realized then that I had found my calling. My whole world changed overnight. I started reading, researching, and speaking with home birth midwives; I went to a midwifery conference. Finally, I said, "This is what I want to do." I did a 180-degree turnaround.

I definitely understand people who want to do it in the hospital, who feel safe in the hospital, but very often that feeling of safety that's in the hospital is a complete illusion. The feeling of safety, "Well, he's a doctor," it doesn't mean you'll have a better result.

Everybody does have to do their research and do what is good for them. I never try to convince anyone to have a home birth. I want people to make an informed choice, and prepare themselves for it, and make their own decisions."

Barbara continues:

I know that when I worked at Hadassah Hospital, I was a very senior midwife, and the doctors I worked with would ask me to come in and deliver their wives. Then I left and became a home birth midwife, and I met one of the doctors whose baby's birth I had attended in the hospital, and he asked me, "Barbara, I have a question. When you go to a home birth, do you bring along equipment?"

I said to him, "You don't know anything about home birth, do you?" and he said, "No."

That's why they think it's crazy. They think I come with nothing. People need to know what we are, our training, the risks involved. They need to know all this.

CHAPTER 12

How to have a Home Birth at the Hospital

Maybe you love the idea of a home birth but don't want to give up the medical technology that's available at the hospital. Is it possible to have a home birth-like experience at a hospital?

The answer is it's possible, but it will take some planning. The first thing to do is to pin down what is important to you. Having a home birth at the hospital means different things to different people. For one mother it means being treated with respect and being a part of the decision-making process. For another mother, it means giving birth without any pain medication and having the freedom to birth in the position that feels right to her. To yet another mother it means having an evidence-based birth where she receives medical care and interventions that have been statistically proven to produce the best outcomes for her and her baby.

After you define what a home birth at the hospital means to you, you can then search for a provider and hospital that will support you. Consider first choosing a hospital whose policies most align with your vision. Realistically, the hospital may have a greater impact on you and your baby's birth experience than the provider you choose. Doctors and midwives are constricted by a hospital's policies and procedures. It, therefore, makes sense to first find a hospital with a more natural approach to child-birth, and then choose one of their providers who shares your vision. A hospital midwife is usually going to be more open to a natural woman-centered birth than an obstetrician, as well as have a lower c-section rate. However, while we can make generalizations, doctors and midwives still have their own individual approaches to childbirth. Some obstetricians are really supportive of natural birth, and some midwives are pseudo-doctors, where they don't offer much labor support and just show up at the end of labor to catch the baby.

One thing you will have to be prepared to do when giving birth at a hospital is advocate for yourself. Many women enter hospital doors feeling like their role in childbirth is to be a "good patient" and follow their health care provider's and nurse's instructions. However, your primary task during labor is to have your baby as safely and smoothly as possible. This includes making your needs known, asking for what you want, and even politely refusing an unnecessary intervention.

In addition, having a doula at a hospital birth is even more important than at a home birth. You are extremely vulnerable during labor and birth, and having someone navigating the system for you and being your voice can make a very big difference in how your birth plays out.

A 2017 Cochrane Review[215] found that having continuous support during labor is consistent with a shorter duration of labor. You also have a lower risk of an assisted vaginal birth or c-section.

The following story illustrates the difference a doula can make during a difficult birth.

Carla's Story

Carla, a 25-year-old first-time mom, had her baby with an obstetrician at a local hospital. She needed the security of knowing there was a NICU and an OR down the hall just in case. Her obstetrician was known to be laid-back when it came to medical interventions and she felt comfortable with him. She chose a highly experienced doula to support her during labor, and when the time came, they went down to the hospital together to labor. Carla's doctor met them there and found Carla was dilated 4 centimeters. Carla labored with her doula, finding relief in different positions and different labor coping techniques.

As the hours passed by, Carla's doctor began addressing the slow progress she was making. Carla's doula asked for more time and really worked with her to help her relax and advance her labor. Carla stepped into the shower and relaxed under the jets of water. Carla's doula continued to advocate for Carla as the baby's heart rate remained steady. Finally, after many hours, Carla was fully dilated and ready to push.

Carla was nearing exhaustion but the doula encouraged and supported her as she was nearly there. Carla's obstetrician instructed her on pushing, and he gently maneuvered her baby out. After hearing Carla's story, more than one person commented if she had not had her doula, she would likely have had a c-section. Carla was so grateful to her doula for believing in her and not giving up.

Carla's doula advocated for her, and with her help, Carla achieved her goal of having a natural birth.

Renske Kuiper[216], a Dutch midwife, explains her stance:

I am not against a hospital birth, because some women will feel more comfortable there, and some should be there for medical reasons, and I'm not against epidurals, but it needs to be your choice, and women should be supported in their own choice.

I compare it to a marathon. Not everybody wants to run a marathon, and that's okay. But if you run a marathon and all along the way people are asking, "You sure you don't want to stop? You don't want to have a drink? You're sure you want to go on?" That's not supportive. You want to have people on the road saying, "You're doing good. Go for it!" and then, if you really want to stop, I'll be there to give you a drink, give you a hug, and say it's okay.

While having supportive people around you during labor impacts your labor positively, having unsupportive people around you can have the opposite effect. Judith Lothian, RN, PhD, published an article[217] in *The Journal of Perinatal Education* in 2004 in which she describes how disturbing a woman during labor can lead to the release of catecholamines[218], also known as stress hormones. Catecholamines may slow down or halt the progression of labor. This is because it puts your body into "fight or flight" mode which counteracts oxytocin release.

What are your options if that happens to you during labor? What if a nurse speaks to you in a way that makes you feel uncomfortable? Maybe they're commenting on your lack of progress, or maybe they keep pressuring you to take an epidural. Every person brings an energy into the room with them. If a person is giving off negative vibes, then it is counterproductive to have them present.

To help prevent this situation, it is best to be proactive from the outset of your hospital stay in establishing rapport with the nursing staff. You can bring along some donuts for them, make small talk, and show an interest in them. In a friendly way, you can explain to them why you prefer to labor without an epidural, why you want to keep your baby skin-to-skin right after birth, and what the birth experience means to you. In addition, explain that as much as you have things you wish for at your birth, you understand that, of course, your safety and your baby's safety are paramount. Your nurse wants to do her job, which is keeping you and your baby safe during the delivery. Showing your respect for their job will motivate them to want to help you achieve your birthing goals. Understanding where they are coming from and alleviating their concerns can go a long way toward building trust and cooperation.

It is possible, though, that the nurse assigned to you may have a difficult personality and be unsupportive of your wishes. As a last resort, know that it is within your rights to request a different nurse.

Another question you may have is what if your health care provider comes by and feels it's time to intervene medically? Hopefully, you have discussed your wishes with them prior to birth, and you are on the same page as to when interventions will be employed.

If you are confused as to why an intervention is needed though, you have the right to ask three simple questions:

1. Is mom okay?
2. Is the baby okay?
3. Can we have more time?

Asking those questions will encourage your provider to take another look at what is going on, and will clarify for everyone if the intervention is truly necessary.

Dr. Marsden Wagner, in his book *Born in the USA*[219], notes there are laws in the United States that require a doctor to obtain informed consent for any procedure. That means your provider must ask your permission before doing any procedure or intervention. That also means you have the right to refuse any intervention. It's your body and your baby. You have every right to advocate for yourself by refusing any interventions you are not comfortable with, or do not see a good reason for. Anything that is done to you should only be done with your consent.

EMT and birth doula April Davis[220], describes the downsides to her hospital birth:

> As much as everything went well, I remember at one point they made me get out of the tub so that my midwife could check me. I was squatting on the end of the table, shaking because I was in transition.
>
> She was checking me, which I'm not in love with, when I heard, "Oh, we haven't started the IV yet–we have to do that," a woman was saying.
>
> I immediately called back a little aggressively, "I don't need this right now. I don't need you talking to me!"
>
> They had me sign paperwork while I was in the tub having a contraction. It was embarrassing. This is one element that hospitals need to improve upon.

In 2009, the *Journal of Perinatal Education* published an article[221] about the abuse, and potential for abuse, of women giving birth in a hospital environment. Women giving birth are in an extremely vulnerable position. Because of this, health care professionals must ensure they obtain express permission before doing an exam or procedure. For example, if a health care provider walks up to a patient and tells them to lie on their back so they can do a vaginal exam, that is not okay. Doctors, midwives, and nurses need to ask for consent before they do a vaginal exam, or any other intervention. If a patient does not consent, then they need to better explain why it is necessary. If the woman continues to refuse, then the health care provider needs to accept that. It is her body and therefore her right to refuse. Hospital personnel may be so bent on doing their "job" that they don't realize their behavior constitutes abuse.

Obstetric violence[222] is unfortunately a reality in hospitals around the world, and occurs more frequently than you might think. Stories[223] are told by women about trauma inflicted on them by doctors and hospital personnel. Women report having interventions and procedures done to them without prior consent. They report being spoken down to, or being pressured or bullied into an intervention that wasn't actually necessary, and even expressly against their wishes.

Dr. Wagner wrote a paper[224] titled, "Fish can't see water: the need to humanize birth." The paper brings to light the importance of health care providers viewing their obstetric patients as human beings who have the right to choose where and how to give birth to their babies. Women know their physical, emotional, and psychological needs more intimately than anyone else around them. Being free to consent or withhold consent for a procedure being done to them is a basic human right.

In 2017, a study[225] was published in *BMC Pregnancy and Childbirth* describing a variety of childbirth situations that are viewed as traumatic by the mother. Women related situations where their providers were perceived as prioritizing their own needs over those of the patient. For example, a provider was overheard commenting on his need to get to an event, while intervening to speed up the birth process. Other situations women reported were providers dismissing the patient's own assessment of her labor progression, providers ignoring symptoms they were describing, and providers ignoring concerns mothers had about their baby. Participants in the study universally reported feeling like their needs and wishes were irrelevant.

A mother's perception[226] of her birth experience impacts the way she recalls it. Feeling unheard and ignored during labor and birth will likely lead a mother to reflect negatively on her experience. Conversely, a complicated delivery where mom was supported emotionally and given autonomy in the decision process, may be less psychologically traumatic[227] than a less complicated delivery where mom was mistreated.

How common is traumatic birth?

About one-third[228] of women who give birth view their experience as traumatic, and around 3 to 4% of women who give birth go on to develop PTSD[229]. Risk factors[230] for PTSD include a complicated delivery where fear for the baby's life was present, difficult interactions with hospital staff during labor, lingering feelings of shame around the birth, feeling a loss of control over their environment, and a lack of social support during labor and birth.

PTSD has long-term consequences[231] for a new mother and her family. These include the development of postpartum depression, negative consequences on mom's relationship with her partner, poor bonding with her baby, and subsequent poor social and emotional development[232] of her baby.

On a positive note, across the United States, hospitals and health care providers are partnering to improve the birth experience for moms. For example, Dr. Neel Shah started Team Birth Project[233], a system stressing open communication between doctors, nurses, and parents, in order to reduce the incidence of c-sections. This was created following an initiative by Adriadne labs[234], developed by Dr. Atul Gawande, with Brigham and Women's Hospital and the Harvard T.H. Chan School of Public Health in Boston.

Team Birth Project puts up a whiteboard in each patient's room that is marked up and split into sections. One section describes and lists the parents' preferences for the birth. The second section is designated "What Happens Next." This section tells parents what will happen next in the birth process, and what the nurse or health care provider will be doing.

Kaiser Health News published an article[235] illustrating what Team Birth Project looks like as it plays out. The article covers a twins' VBAC birth that took place at South Shore Hospital in Weymouth, Massachusetts in August 2018. It was very important to the parents that every effort be made to avoid a c-section. The hospital made its best effort to honor the parents' request, despite the fact that the second of the twins was not in an optimal position for birth. The second twin was in a side lying, also known as transverse position. The mom agreed to receive an epidural and deliver her babies in the operating room. This way, if a c-section was required it could happen immediately. The parents were kept updated throughout labor, with the nurses and doctors communicating openly with them. Both babies were delivered vaginally, and a c-section was successfully avoided. The twins' parents commented after the birth that being included in the decision-making process gave them a strong feeling of trust in their providers. They knew they were doing everything they could to honor their wishes around the birth of their twins.

Another important initiative in improving birth is the organization Evidence Based Birth[236]. Evidence Based Birth was started by Rebecca Dekker, RN, PhD, after she had a difficult experience delivering her first baby at a planned hospital birth. Rebecca subsequently used her background in nursing and medical research to determine if the hospital practices she experienced had any merit to them. Rebecca found that many of the hospital's protocols and procedures she experienced were not evidence-based. The realization that women around the country, and around the world, were being subjected to interventions that were not only unhelpful, but even harmful, led her to start Evidence Based Birth. Evidence Based Birth is an organization and a movement that educates and empowers women, medical students, doctors, nurses, and birth workers on best birth practices. Rebecca's organization can be found at evidencebasedbirth.com. It provides research articles on common obstetric practices, providing hard data on their effectiveness and outcomes. It is a great resource for anyone interested in learning more about best birth practices.

Birthing in a hospital that supports evidence-based care will give you and your baby a better birth experience with better outcomes.

An example of an evidence-based practice hospitals are adopting is delayed cord clamping. The practice of early cord clamping, which is when the cord is clamped and cut right away at birth, started in the 1960s. It was believed to reduce the incidence of postpartum hemorrhage. This thinking has since been disproven[237]. Studies show that delaying cord clamping, which is waiting a few minutes after birth before cutting the cord, allows up to 30% more oxygen and nutrient rich blood to flow to the baby.

In January of 2017, ACOG released a statement[238] recommending obstetricians delay cord clamping for all babies, due to the multiple benefits it provides for them. A major benefit is the extra iron stores the baby receives in the cord blood. Iron is important for brain development, as well as preventing iron deficiency anemia. Cord blood also contains stem cells and immunoglobulins that aid in tissue repair. The only drawback to delayed cord clamping appears to be a slightly increased risk for jaundice to the newborn due to the extra blood volume.

The World Health Organization (WHO) supports the practice of delayed cord clamping at birth[239], citing "improved maternal and infant health and nutrition outcomes."

Another evidence-based birth practice recommended by WHO in 2018[240] is ensuring the opportunity for mother and baby to have skin-to-skin contact right after birth. Traditionally, hospitals remove babies from their mothers at birth and place them under warming lights to bring up their body temperature. When providing skin-to-skin contact, the baby is placed on its mother's chest in just a diaper, with a blanket to cover.

The *Journal of Perinatal Education*[241] describes the benefits of keeping mother and baby together after the baby is born. At birth, mothers and babies have high levels of oxytocin, which makes it the perfect time for bonding, as well as a good time to initiate breastfeeding. Skin-to-skin contact at birth also reduces depression[242] and anxiety in mothers in the first week after birth.

An evidence-based practice some hospitals are instituting is delaying a newborn's first bath. In 2016, the Sherman Hospital[243] in Illinois instituted a policy of waiting 14 hours from the time a baby is born before it receives its first bath. After a month of following this policy, they reviewed the rates of hypothermia (low body temperature), hypoglycemia (low blood sugar), and breastfeeding. They compared the rates after the change was implemented to the rates before the change was implemented. The hospital found that when they delayed newborns' first baths, newborn hypothermia rates dropped from 29% to 14%, newborn hypoglycemia rates fell from 21% to 7%, and breastfeeding rates increased from 51% to 78%.

What is it about delaying a newborns' first bath that proves so beneficial? Newborns are born with a special substance, vernix, that is produced by the baby during the third trimester. Vernix[244] is a white sticky, cheesy layer that covers the baby's skin. Physiologically, when we are cold, our bodies burn up sugar trying to keep us warm. Newborns, too, will expend a lot of energy to keep warm, and therefore keeping vernix on their skin as an extra layer of insulation is very beneficial for them. Because they don't burn so much energy trying to warm themselves, they have more energy to engage with their mother and begin breastfeeding. Another benefit of vernix is that is provides an extra layer of protection from bacteria[245].

Sherman Hospital is one of many hospitals around the country, and around the world, that is successfully adopting evidence-based practices in their facilities. They are committed to providing a supportive environment for new mothers, with experienced nurses available to guide new parents in caring for their newborns. For first-time parents, especially, it is really helpful having a nurse show you how to bathe your baby, show you how to change your baby's diaper, help you with breastfeeding, and answer any questions you may have. Many hospitals even have lactation consultants available for specialized breastfeeding help, which can be incredibly valuable.

Pediatricians are available on-site, or on call, if you have a question and want someone to see your baby right away. Newborn hearing screenings are usually done at the hospital as well.

Some hospitals will offer you the option of keeping your baby in the newborn nursery overnight, so you can get some rest before going home. It is comforting to know there is a nurse keeping watch over your baby while you sleep.

Samantha's Story

Samantha and her husband spent two days after the birth of her baby soaking up all the information she needed to care for her baby at home.

Diapering was a whole lesson on its own. Samantha and her husband had never cared for a newborn before as this was the first baby born into either of their families in decades.

Samantha learned how to breastfeed, although she sometimes received conflicting advice about it. Some nurses recommended nursing on demand and some told her she must schedule her baby. The lactation consultants assisted her with the latch which was really helpful, and they recommended creams to help with her sore nipples.

Samantha learned how to swaddle her baby to help him sleep better.

By the time they were discharged home, Samantha and her husband felt comfortable they had the information they needed to care for their baby.

Birthing Centers

Birthing centers are an alternative setting to a hospital or home birth. Birth centers endeavor to create a more homey atmosphere than you might find at a hospital, and are supportive of natural birth. Birthing centers do not offer epidurals but support natural, drug-free options for labor support. Birthing centers have a shorter postpartum stay than a hospital, usually under 24 hours. Like at a home birth, a hospital transfer is required for any complications during labor or birth.

Women choose birthing centers for their natural approach. A study[246] done in the United States found that the c-section rate for women giving birth at a birthing center is 6%, which is significantly lower than the c-section rate at hospital births.

The two kinds of birthing centers you will find are free-standing and hospital-based. Free-standing birth centers are midwife-led and may or may not be affiliated with a hospital.

Hospital-based birthing centers are run by hospitals and cater to women who prefer a natural, unmedicated birth. Some parents feel they have the best of both worlds with the ability to labor in a more natural setting, along with the security of having doctors and an operating room a few minutes away.

Some birth centers are even located adjacent to a hospital, so that there is virtually no travel time if a hospital is needed. However, hospital-based birthing centers may be more restricted with what they can allow, as they still have to follow hospital policies. If a birthing center birth sounds interesting to you, call and schedule a visit to see if it is the right birth setting for you.

CHAPTER 13

What Steps Can You Take to Improve Your Birth Experience?

Childbirth is a high stakes situation with many unknowns. You want to give your baby the best possible start, and you yourself want to be in the best possible state to nurture and care for your baby.

Annie Duke, in her book *Thinking in Bets*[247], discusses how to make a decision when you don't have all the facts. Childbirth is a prime example of a situation where you are making critical decisions without having all the facts. Even a very experienced obstetrician or midwife cannot tell you how your birth will unfold. There are two planning strategies you can employ to lower the risks around your birth. The first strategy is backcasting, and the second is carrying out a premortem.

Backcasting

Backcasting is a strategy where you define your desired outcome in clear detail. You then work backward, planning all the steps you need to take that will get you to your desired outcome.

When it comes to childbirth, your desired outcome is holding a healthy baby in your arms while basking in the afterglow of an empowering birth experience. You gave birth in an atmosphere of love and support.

How did you get to that point? What did you need to do to make that happen? What kind of planning goes into having a beautiful and safe birth?

The first step to making that happen is by putting together a stellar birth team. Begin by doing your research and speaking to women in your community about their birth experiences with different providers. You can also Google birth providers in your area for information about them. Next, draw up a shortlist of providers whose birthing styles are in sync with what you are looking for, and set up meetings with them to discuss what they can offer you.

When you meet a prospective home birth midwife, be prepared with questions for them. You can download and print a free comprehensive list of interview questions at www.homebirthmom. com.

Some sample questions include:
- What are your qualifications?
- What is your philosophy on home birth?
- How long have you been practicing?
- What criteria does a woman need to meet in order to have a home birth with you?

- Do you provide labor support?
- Do you bring along any support professionals when you attend a home birth?
- Will you have another licensed professional with you for the birth?
- What are your feelings about transferring to a hospital if there are problems during labor? For what kind of problems would you transfer a woman to the hospital?
- What emergency equipment do you bring to a home birth?
- Have you ever lost a mother or a baby at a delivery?

When interviewing a midwife or a doctor for a hospital birth, asking open-ended questions will give you a feel for their approach. For example, if you ask them if they support natural birth, almost every birth professional will say yes. However, asking them, "What does a natural birth look like to you?" will give you better insight into what your birth experience will look like under their care.

Another technique to determining a provider's philosophy is explaining your birth plan while carefully gauging their reaction to it. Are they fully supportive of your plan, or do they seem uncomfortable with it?

Other sample questions include:

- How do you typically manage your patient's labor? How does the birth process unfold when your patient gets to the hospital?
- How do you feel about patients bringing a doula to the birth?
- When would EFM be needed?
- At what point would you not allow a patient in labor and delivery to eat or drink?
- What would be a reason for an induction?
- What is your c-section rate?

- In what situations would a c-section be necessary?
- In what situations do you perform an episiotomy? How often does that happen?
- What other positions are you open to delivering a baby in, besides the lithotomy position?
- Who is your back up doctor? Will I get to meet him or her?
- Have you ever done delayed cord clamping?
- How much time will I have with my baby in the immediate time after birth?

You should feel comfortable with your provider's personality, attitude towards birth, level of expertise, and safety record.

Choosing a doula follows a similar process. Research doulas in your area through speaking with other moms. Listen to their birth stories to hear how their doulas reacted and supported them throughout labor and birth. Meet with several birth doulas to determine who is the best fit for you and your partner.

You may also choose to attend childbirth education classes, such as hypnobirthing[248] or evidence based birthing class[249].

Closer to your due date you may look into purchasing or renting a birth tub, birthing ball or peanut ball. There are many other labor coping techniques you can look into that will help you labor comfortably, without pain medication.

Premortem

In Chapter 6 of her book *Thinking in Bets*[250], Duke describes doing a premortem in order to help you make the best decision. A premortem is like backcasting, except you're thinking of all of the things that could go wrong and then planning how you would respond to those scenarios. It essentially ensures you don't miss anything, and that you are more realistic about the probabilities and outcomes of your choices. It also gives you tools to address any glitches that may come up.

Duke writes in her book, "Being able to respond to the changing future is a good thing; being surprised by the changing future is not. Scenario planning makes us nimbler because we've considered and are prepared for a wider variety of possible futures."

Imagining a variety of possible situations that may occur during labor and childbirth will enable you to anticipate and plan for any eventuality. Better planning produces a more realistic view of the unpredictability of childbirth. Discussing it in advance with your partner and health care provider will ensure you are prepared for difficult decisions.

Possible scenarios to plan for include:

> At what point would you want an epidural? You may also want to consider what you would do if the anesthesiologist who comes in to start the epidural seems really young and unpracticed.

> What if your health care provider feels a c-section is warranted? What are your parameters for agreeing to one?

> What if you are at the hospital and your birth plan for the immediate postpartum period is not being honored? For example, you wanted to have your baby skin-to-skin and breastfeed right away, but the nurse insists on doing her newborn assessment and wants to keep your baby under a warmer for several minutes afterwards. What if you refuse administering erythromycin eye gel and a vitamin k shot to your newborn, but the nurse tells you it's the hospital's protocol and you don't have a choice? What would you be willing to compromise on?

Doing a premortem helps prevent a traumatic birth. Birth trauma[251] stems from feeling like a victim of circumstances. Preparing for, and thinking about, a variety of scenarios provides you with the tools you need to help avoid a traumatic birth, or at least lessen the trauma of a difficult situation.

A scenario which commonly occurs at planned home births is when the midwife feels transferring to the hospital is the right decision. That can be traumatic if you had your heart set on a home birth. Knowing in advance that a transfer to hospital is likely, can help you feel prepared if it comes to pass.

This occurred to Yehudit Debrova[252], a home birth mom, as she describes in an interview: "With home birth, if I could change something, I would tell a mother a transfer is possible, and there should be a just-in-case hospital bag packed with some clothes and toiletries.

I had to go the hospital with not much warning and I didn't have much with me in the hospital. It would have made a difficult situation easier if I would have been prepared for it."

At a home birth, the likelihood of a transfer to the hospital is around 10% for a woman who has previously given birth and higher for a woman who's having her first baby. A planned home birth may turn into a hospital birth for a number of reasons. A study was published in *BMC Pregnancy and Childbirth* in 2014 titled "Transfer to hospital in planned home births: a Systematic Review." This research project gathered 15 studies on planned home births from a variety of countries that included Australia, Canada, USA, UK, Sweden, Norway, Denmark, and the Netherlands for a total of 215,257 births studied.

The percentage of planned home births that turned into hospital births varied from 9.9% to 31.9% across the studies. The most common indication for hospital transfer was labor dystocia (prolonged labor). This occurred in 5.1% to 9.8% of all women planning home births. Transferring for fetal distress ranged from 1.0% to 3.6%. After the birth, transfer for postpartum hemorrhage ranged from 0% to 0.2%. Transfer for respiratory problems in the infant ranged from 0.3% to 1.4%.

It's important to ask a midwife about her hospital transfer rate, as hospital transfer rates are a sign of a cautious, safe midwife. Israeli midwife Mindy Levy[253] explains:

> My overall transfer rate is 14%. Very often it is intuitive. I just get a bad feeling that things are not progressing well and that home is no longer the right place to be.
> Something comes along, either meconium staining or there's a problem with the baby's heartbeat, or there's some bleeding, or a woman feels like she can't go on and she needs an epidural. I do not like emergency transfers. I prefer to transfer way before the emergency occurs.

Mindy elaborates:

> My c-section rate is 4%. So a lot of those transfers do not end up in c-sections. A lot of those transfers end up normal vaginal births. The chance of ending up with a c-section when having a home birth is very low…If I examine the woman and the cervix is rigid, that's a bad sign. Instead of everything being soft, and the baby's head coming down, the cervix thinning out, and the head getting lower, all of a sudden, it goes in the other direction. It's an internal sign that something's wrong, that the uterus is not in a good place.

When asked why that would happen, Mindy responds, "It may not necessarily be emotional. It could be the head was coming down at a bad angle, and there was no progress, and she was just getting really, really tired. The resulting fatigue then made her stressed."

Mindy explains what happens when she gets to the hospital, "Very often the woman will take an epidural, she'll relax and rest, and then the cervix will soften up again."

Many women fear what would happen if they needed an emergency c-section at a planned home birth. Ruthie Pearlman[254], home birth doula, observes:

> A lot of people talk about their emergency c-section.
>
> It is actually rare for a true emergency c-section.
>
> What usually happens is the doctor will see the way labor is progressing and can see this is going down a road that if it were to continue we would want to not have a bad outcome so we're going to step in now and do a c-section to prevent that.
>
> So there's time. They prep the OR. They give you IV fluids. Give you papers to sign.
>
> Keeping that in mind, home birth midwives are listening to the baby and checking vitals and doing all the things they need to do, so it is not like, "We need to go to the hospital right this second because the baby's in distress."
>
> They'll say, "Oh we're noticing the baby's having some heart decelerations. Your color doesn't look great. We're going to the hospital now before anything becomes an emergency crisis."
>
> So a hospital transfer is always possible at a home birth and it does happen. You can always go to a hospital if you need to.
>
> It's good to plan which hospital you would transfer to if needed while you're still pregnant.
>
> It's even better if you have a midwife who has privileges there and you're not just coming in through the emergency room.

Really, in 95% of situations, midwives know what to do and are prepared for it.

Having a plan in case you need to be transferred to the hospital during labor is a good idea. April Davis[255], a home birth mom, prepared for a hospital birth and a home birth by having shared care. This way, if she needed to be in the hospital for her birth, she had a care provider for her there. This is her story.

April's Story

I have hyperemesis gravidarum where I can't keep food down for nine months, so it was kind of hard. This was my third and last and by far worst pregnancy, and I was actually on a PICC line (IV) for a lot of my pregnancy.

I went through my pregnancy just trying to keep fluid inside me.

I knew going into it that while I wanted a home birth, if I can't get my iron level where it needs to be, I can't deliver at home, and if I'm still this sick, then I can't deliver at home.

I actually did shared care, so I saw a hospital midwife and I also saw Cyndi, the home birth midwife that I worked for. So I visited with both of them throughout my entire pregnancy and was cared for by both of them and then toward the end, my iron levels were where they were supposed to be and I was doing pretty good, so we decided let's move ahead with home birth, but if things got sketchy, we'd switch back over.

I had a place to land if I needed to go back into the medical system.

I start getting contractions the minute my third trimester hits, so I had been contracting for forever and they were getting worse and worse and I wasn't due until mid-January.

After Christmas, I decided it was time to have Cyndi do a stretch and sweep to get this baby out. I couldn't do another night with contractions and throwing up, and I was ready to quit and be done!

I woke up on the 28th of December and was throwing up and I called my midwife and told her I can't be pregnant anymore. So she said, "Okay, I'll come over."

I just wish people could know how great it is to have a medical provider come over to your home and not have to get into a car.

She came over, checked me, and said, "You're sitting on a 5 still."

I had been at a 5 for a couple of days at that point. She said she could do a little stretch and sweep and let's see if we could get things rolling.

She was fairly aggressive with the stretch and sweep.

I had already lost my mucus plug at that point. I had some good signs of labor happening.

I sat on a bouncy ball for 2 hours, and she watched me and nothing happened so she went home.

She said, "Go on a walk. If 3 o'clock in the afternoon rolls around, you go to bed and you stay in bed."

It was 2:30.

I put on my leggings, and I had my daughter lace up my athletic shoes. We were going for a WALK.

I got to the end of my driveway, and I had this huge gush of fluid, and I thought my water had finally broke.

I was so happy.

I go inside and it's not my water, it's blood.

I called my midwife and she said she'll be there in a minute. My husband came home. By the time she got to my house 5 minutes later I was already having good contractions.

She checked me, checked on the baby, did all of the vitals, and said we looked fine and probably just disrupted a lot when she did the stretch and sweep, so she said, "Let's move forward, but if you keep bleeding like this, we might go in."

So we filled up the tub and I hopped into it, and my husband hopped in and within a half hour after that, I was pushing. He was born just before 5 o'clock.

The birth was a dream. I felt so uninhibited. I knew everyone there, and I was surrounded by so much love and support.

I was able to just let everything open and go and just have him.

The sad thing is women don't believe me. They don't believe me when I tell them this. They think it's just not possible.

My labor probably would have been longer if I would have been in the hospital. I think some of the shortness of it and the smoothness of things moving along was because I was comfortable. I was at home. I was in my safe space. I was in my bubble.

It was amazing.

I was able to catch my baby.

It went really well.

I bled afterwards as my placenta didn't come, so my midwife had to go in and get it, and that was not my favorite, but other than that, it was fantastic.

April ended up having the home birth she dreamed about, but she made plans in case Plan A didn't work out. Some midwives have privileges at the local hospital, which means they can continue caring for you at the hospital if you were transferred. Some midwives partner with an obstetrician that would be available to medically intervene, as well as perform a c-section if needed.

Some midwives will ask their client to sign a contract before agreeing to take them on. The contract includes what the midwife offers the client, and what the client agrees to adhere to, when working with the midwife. Below, you can read a sample contract.

The Midwifery Services, LLC, agrees to:

- Determine the client's eligibility for a home birth through review of medical history, physical examination findings, lab results, and existing support systems.

- Provide the client with prenatal care and guidance through-out pregnancy, labor, birth, and postpartum as long as pregnancy remains normal as defined by the midwives' protocols.
- Provide on-going evaluation throughout pregnancy, labor, birth and the postpartum period with careful attention to signs of normalcy or deviation from normal. All findings will be discussed openly with the client.
- Provide information regarding procedures, treatments, and medications to enable the client to make informed choices regarding the course of her pregnancy, labor and birth.
- Provide 24-hour on-call service for the client during her pregnancy and childbirth. Coverage from another licensed midwife will be provided in the event of planned time off, illness or emergency. The staff will notify the client in the event of substitute midwife coverage during your window of potential delivery dates.
- Provide one prenatal home visit at 36 weeks.
- Provide care during labor and birth when labor starts after 37 weeks of pregnancy and before 42 weeks.
- Provide at least one postpartum home visit and two postpartum office visits.
- Provide a trained birth assistant to be present at the birth.
- Refer the client to medical services if any abnormal condition appears, with discharge to another care provider if appropriate.
- If hospitalization becomes necessary during labor, birth, or the immediate postpartum period, the client's records will accompany her and will be made available to the consulting physician and medical staff. The client's transport would take place according to her personalized emergency care plan. The attending midwife would accompany her to the hospital, where she would give report to the attending medical staff,

unless her services were simultaneously required by another client for birthing care. Whenever possible, the midwife will stay with the mother until after the birth and breastfeeding is established.

- In choosing to birth at home, the Client knowingly accept responsibility for the labor and birth. The Client realizes that no matter how carefully they are assessed, unforeseen events may arise, resulting in poor outcome. Although pregnancy and birth are natural physiologic processes, certain medical conditions may arise necessitating consultation, collaboration, or transfer of care from Midwifery Services, LLC to that of a nurse midwife or physician in a hospital. Depending on the reason, transfer may be considered emergent or non-emergent and may be due to maternal, fetal, or newborn indications.

- The Client is aware that emergencies occurring in the home are handled in a medically supportive fashion until transfer to the hospital is accomplished. The Client agrees to transfer mother and/or infant to physician management and hospital care if the course of pregnancy, birth, or the postpartum period becomes medically complicated and the midwife determines that rendering care to the Client is outside of her scope or available resources. Whenever possible, the decisions regarding such transfers will be made jointly by Clients, the midwife, and the consulting providers. Clients understand, however, that a situation may arise where Clients must accept the judgment of the midwife and proceed accordingly.

- Arrange for an adult other than the primary support person to be responsible for any small children that will be present at the time of labor and birth.

- Actively promote a healthy pregnancy by maintaining excellent nutrition and sound health practices, including regular exercise, avoiding caffeine, tobacco, alcohol, and other drugs and keeping her scheduled prenatal appointments.

- Have requested birth kit supplies ready by 36 weeks of pregnancy.
- Agree to transfer mother or baby to the hospital if the midwife detects problems that can be managed appropriately only in the hospital.
- Clients willingly accept the risks associated with home birth, and hereby consent to the care provided by Midwifery Services, LLC. Clients hereby release Midwifery Services, LLC, the midwives, and the midwifery assistants from all liability arising from acts or omissions on their part while functioning according to their practice guidelines. Clients further acknowledge that the midwife and midwifery assistants of Midwifery Services, LLC are not covered by medical malpractice, errors, and omission insurance.

This sample contract is a good guideline of what a home birth midwife expects from her client, as well as what you'd be agreeing to if you plan a home birth.

You may feel comfortable planning a home birth, but are hesitating because you know your family would disapprove. Some women dream about having a home birth, but ultimately choose to birth with an obstetrician in the hospital because their family discourages them from having one Batsheva Nagel, a home birth mom, relates in an interview.

> My husband has always been supportive of my decision of where to birth our babies as he says: "Whatever you want. You're the one having the baby."
> My Mom was pretty supportive. I knew my sisters would be a very skeptical as they are skeptical with things that are not common practice so I knew that telling them was going to be

a little hard for me. So I just said: "Listen I love you guys and I value your opinion. I'm doing what I think is best for me and my family and it's a safe situation with an experienced midwife who's been with me from the beginning."

They said: "You're right we don't necessarily agree but we trust your judgement and everything should just go smoothly." So that was nice as I went into it I felt everyone was sort of on board.

My mother-in-law just told my husband's grandmother after the fact that it all happened too fast and we didn't make it to the hospital, which is actually in the end what happened and I wouldn't have made it to the hospital.

Sometimes your family doesn't have much prior knowledge about home birth, but they are nevertheless open-minded about it. When Sarah Lewis[256] was asked how her family reacted to the news that she was planning a home birth, she related, "They didn't give me a hard time, but they were a little unsure about it. They trusted me to do what was right, but they weren't so familiar with the concept of a home birth, so they had to adjust to the idea."

Sarah Lewis continues:

I'm not actually such a home birth advocate.

I know for myself that I can do it.

I prefer it because I have confidence in myself and my body and its abilities.

But I do wish people would know it is not a dangerous, risky, careless, irresponsible thing to do. I get that a lot, and I don't like talking about it for that reason because I get a lot of backlash.

I usually feel out other mothers before being open about it.
You can tell other mothers who think it's cool or have done
it or are interested in having one.

And you can tell other mothers who would never do it in
a million years and who are totally judging you and I won't
start up a conversation with them about it.

Having to contend with family and friends who think home birth
is a terrible idea can be stressful.

Jennifer Griffin[257] speaks about this in an interview, "My
mother was actually equally terrified by the fourth home birth
as the first, calling every day before I was due, freaking out,
and I always said that she couldn't know when I was in labor
because I didn't want her negative energy affecting me. She
was so concerned, and I had already done this successfully
three times, but it really scared her that I was doing this."

Leah Marinelli, CNM, a home birth midwife who wants people
to understand the risks involved in a planned home birth, explicitly
stated in an interview:[258] "Home birth is not for everyone. You
have to know yourself. You have to know what criticism you might
have to face if things don't go exactly perfectly. It's accepting
responsibility in a culture that is not home birth oriented."

Even if you are a good candidate for a home birth, if you are
sensitive to criticism, you may choose to give birth in the hospital
due to the backlash you know you'll face for your decision. Dealing
with family member's disapproval and distress over your decision
may not be worth the negative effect it will have on you and your
pregnancy.

On the other hand, you may be able to strengthen your resolve
in the face of criticism by reminding yourself, and educating
your family members, that competent home birth midwives are

tuned in to mom and baby and can foresee complications. They recognize early signs that labor is not progressing adequately and will transport to the hospital, erring on the side of caution every time.

Real emergencies rarely pop up without early warning signs, and midwives use those early warning signs to move mom to the hospital where mom will be closer to the operating room just in case it is needed.

At a home birth, midwives will bring at least one other medical support person in order to have one health care professional focused solely on mom and one solely on baby.

Midwives are trained in newborn resuscitation and newborn care. That is why a pediatrician does not need to see your baby immediately after birth. Midwives check the heart and lungs, Apgar scores, newborn reflexes, and vital signs.

It may be worth having a conversation about your desire for a home birth with your family members whose opinion is important to you. You can even give them this book to read. Many people don't know much about home birth, and don't realize how safe it can be.

What if you're at a point where your hospital birth is all set up and you are now having second thoughts?

Would switching providers work for you?

I don't know.

But you need to ask yourself what you have to lose by looking into alternative options. Many women have hospital births and that works for them. But if you are now feeling unsure about your plans, it's definitely worth looking into alternative options for the peace of mind it brings knowing you are making the decision that's right for you. Switching providers and birth settings late in your pregnancy is doable, and it may be the decision that's right for you.

In Conclusion

I hope this book gave you some clarity as you decide on the place that's right for you to birth your baby. Whether you choose to give birth in the hospital, at home, or at a birthing center, the important thing is that you have the knowledge and information to plan a safe and supportive birth.

Once you've made your decision, remember that your birth experience will unfold as it was meant to. Plan your birth as best you can and then enjoy the ride. It is an adventure you and your baby will embark on together.

I'd like to leave you with a quote from Marie Mongan, of *Hypnobirthing*[259]:

"My dream is that every woman, everywhere, will know the joy of a truly safe, comfortable, and satisfying birthing for herself and her baby."

Good luck with your decision and congratulations!

Afterword

Thank you so much for taking the time to read this book. If you have any questions, please reach out to me at ihomebirthmom@gmail.com and I will do my best to answer you.

To read the interviews in full, or for bonus content, like a free printable list of interview questions for a prospective midwife, go to www.homebirthmom.com

Notes

1 Lothian, Judith A. "Being safe: Making the decision to have a planned home birth in the United States." *Journal of Clinical Ethic, Volume 24, no. 3, 2013, pp.* 266-275.

2 Lothian, Judith A. *Giving Birth with Confidence, Official Lamaze Guide. New York, De Capo Press, 2013.*

3 Lothian, Judith A. "Do Not Disturb: The Importance of Privacy in Labor." *Journal of Perinatal Education*, vol. 13, no. 3, 2004 https://10.1624/105812404X1707.

4 Pirdel, Manizheh, and Leila Pirdel. "Perceived Environmental Stressors and Pain Perception During Labor Among Primiparous and Multiparous Women." *Journal of Reproduction & Infertility,* vol. 10, no. 3, 2009, pp. 217-23.

5 Dahlen, Hannah. "Interview with Professor Hannah Dahlen, Australian Home Birth Midwife." *Home Birth Mom*, 2019, http://homebirthmom.com/interview-with-professor-hannah-dahlen-australian-home-birth-midwife/.

6 Shiel, William. "Medical Definition of Nosocomial." *MedicineNet*, 2018, https://www.medicinenet.com/script/main/art.asp?articlekey=4590.

7 Sanchini, A, et al. "Outbreak of skin and soft tissue infections in a hospital newborn nursery in Italy due to community-acquired methicillin-resistant Staphylococcus aureus USA300 clone." *Journal of Hospital Infection*, vol. 83, no. 1, November 16, 2012, pp. 36 – 40, https://doi.org/10.1016/j.jhin.2012.09.017.

8 Oaklander, Mandy. "Your Home is Covered in Bacteria." *Time*, August 19, 2014, https://time.com/3209387/house-germs-microbes/.

9 Marinelli, Leah. "Interview with Home Birth Midwife Leah Marinelli." *Home Birth Mom*, 2018, http://homebirthmom.com/interview-with-homebirth-midwife-leah-marinelli/.

10 Groopman, Jerome and Pamela Hartzband. *Your Medical Mind: How to Decide What is Right for You.* The Penguin Press, 2011.

11 Brusie, Chaunie. "Cervix Dilation Chart: The Stages of Labor." *Healthline*, updated on July 8, 2020, https://www.healthline.com/health/pregnancy/cervix-dilation-chart.

12 Heine, Merete, et al. "An In Vitro Study of Antibacterial Properties of the Cervical Mucus Plug in Pregnancy." *American Journal of Obstetrics & Gynecology*, vol. 185, no. 3863, pp. 586-592.

13 "Labor and Delivery, Postpartum Care." *Mayo Clinic,* 2020, https://www.mayoclinic.org/healthy-lifestyle/labor-and-delivery/multimedia/cervical-effacement-and-dilation/img-20006991.

14 Olza, Ibone, et al. "Birth as a neuro-psycho-social event: An integrative model of maternal experiences and their relation to neurohormonal events during childbirth." PLOS ONE, July 28, 2020. *https://doi.org/10.1371/journal.pone.0230992*

15 World Health Organization. "WHO recommendation on definitions of the latent and active first stages of labour." *The WHO Reproductive Healthy Library*, 2018, https://extranet.who.int/rhl/topics/preconception-pregnancy-childbirth-and-postpartum-care/care-during-childbirth/care-during-labour-1st-stage/who-recommendation-definitions-latent-and-active-first-stages-labour-0.

16 Kay, Carolyn. "Cervix Dilation Chart: The Stages of Labor." *Healthline*, 2020, https://www.healthline.com/health/pregnancy/cervix-dilation-chart#stage-1.

17 Molly. "The Rest and Be Thankful Stage." *Talk Birth,* 2012, https://talkbirth.me/2012/02/26/the-rest-and-be-thankful-stage/amp/.

18 "Apgar Score." *MedlinePlus,* 2020, https://medlineplus.gov/ency/article/003402.htm.

19 Speller, Jess. "Placental Development." *TeachMePhysiology,* 2020, https://teachmephysiology.com/reproductive-system/pregnancy/placental-development/.

20 Engel, Yetty. "Interview with Mrs. Yetty Engel, CM." *Home Birth Mom,* 2018, http://homebirthmom.com/yetty-engel-homebirth-midwife/.

21 Levy, Mindy. "Interview with Home Birth Midwife Mindy Levy." *Home Birth Mom*, 2018, http://homebirthmom.com/interview-with-homebirth-midwife-mindy-levy/.

22 Cassidy, Tina. *Birth: The Surprising History of How We Are Born.* Atlantic Monthly Press, 2006, pp.131-158.

23 Leavitt, Judith W. "Joseph B. DeLee and the Practice of Preventive Obstetrics." *AJPH*, vol. 78, no. 10, October 1988, https://ajph.aphapublications.org/doi/pdf/10.2105/AJPH.78.10.1353.

24 Dick-Read, Grantly. *Childbirth Without Fear: The Principles and Practices of Natural Childbirth.* London, Heinemann Medical Books, 1951.

25 Lamaze, F. *Painless Childbirth.* London, Burke, 1958.

26 Bradley, R. "Fathers' Presence in Delivery Rooms." *Psychosomatics*, vol. 3, 1962, pp. 474-479, https://10.1016/s0033-3182(62)72633-2.

27 Lawrence, Annemarie, et al. "Maternal positions and mobility during first stage labour." *The Cochrane Database of Systematic Reviews*, vol. 2, CD003934, 15 Apr. 2009, https://10.1002/14651858.CD003934.pub2.

28 Boyle, Annelee, et al. "Primary Cesarean Delivery in the United States." *Obstetrics and Gynecology,* vol. 122, no. 1, 2013, pp. 33-40, https://10.1097/AOG.0b013e3182952242.

29 Friedlander, Krystina. "A better way to give birth." *CNN,* May 11, 2015, https://www.cnn.com/2015/05/10/opinions/friedlander-midwife-mothers-day/?no-st=9999999999.

30 Kozhimannil, Katy Backes, et al. "Cesarean Delivery Rates Vary 10-fold Among US Hospitals; Reducing Variation May Address Quality, Cost Issues." *Health Affairs (Project Hope),* vol. 32, no. 3, 2013, pp. 527-35, https://10.1377/hlthaff.2012.1030.

31 Almendrala, Anna. "U.S. C-Section Rate is Double What WHO Recommends." *Huffpost,* April 14, 2015, https://www.huffpost.com/entry/c-section-rate-recommendation_n_7058954.

32 World Health Organization. *WHO Statement on Caesarean Section Rates.* Geneva, Switzerland, 2015.

33 Weule, Genelle. "The countries where more than half of babies are delivered via caesarean." *ABC News,* October 14, 2018.

34 Caughey, Aaron B., et al. "Safe Prevention of the Primary Cesarean Delivery." *ACOG,* March 2014, https://www.acog.org:443/en/Clinical/Clinical Guidance/Obstetric Care Consensus/Articles/2014/03/Safe Prevention of the Primary Cesarean Delivery.

35 Shah, Neel. "Are hospitals the safest place for healthy women to have babies? An obstetrician thinks twice." *The Conversation,* June 3, 2015, https://theconversation.com/are-hospitals-the-safest-place-for-healthy-women-to-have-babies-an-obstetrician-thinks-twice-42654.

36 Alexander, James M., et al. "Fetal injury associated with cesarean delivery." *Obstetrics and Gynecology,* vol. 108, no. 4, 2006, pp. 885-90, https://10.1097/01.AOG.0000237116.72011.f3.

37 Belluz, Julia. "Californian decided it was tires of women bleeding to death." *Vox*, December 4, 2017, https://www.vox.com/science-and-health/2017/6/29/15830970/women-health-care-maternal-mortality-rate.

38 Almendrala, Anna. "U.S. C-Section Rate is Double What WHO Recommends." *Huffpost*, April 14, 2015, https://www.huffpost.com/entry/c-section-rate-recommendation_n_7058954.

39 Belluz, Julia. "Californian decided it was tires of women bleeding to death." *Vox*, December 4, 2017, https://www.vox.com/science-and-health/2017/6/29/15830970/women-health-care-maternal-mortality-rate.

40 Cooper, Anne Colleen. "The Rate of Placenta Accreta and Previous Exposure to Uterine Surgery." *Yale Medicine Thesis Digital Library,* 2012, pp. 1702, http://elischolar.library.yale.edu/ymtdl/1702.

41 Ibid.

42 Khokhar, R.S., et al. "Placenta accreta and anesthesia: A multidisciplinary approach." *Saudi Journal of Anaesthesia,* vol. 10, no. 3, 2016, pp. 332-4, https://10.4103/1658-354X.174913.

43 Love, Douglass. "Consumer Reports Analysis: Most U.S. Hospitals' C-Section Rates Exceeding National Targets." *Consumer Reports*, May 5, 2017. https://www.consumerreports.org/media-room/press-releases/2017/05/consumer_reports_analysis_most_us_hospitals_csection_rates_exceeding_national_targets/.

44 Jena, Anupam B., et al. "Physician spending and subsequent risk of malpractice claims: observational study." *BMJ*, 2015, pp. 351.

45 Sartwelle, T.P., et al. "Fetal Monitoring, Cerebral Palsy Litigation, and Bioethics: The Evils in Pandora's Box." *Journal of Pediatric Care*, vol. 2, no. 2, 2016, https://10.21767/2471-805X.100014.

46 Caughey, Aaron B., et al. "Obstetric Care Consensus No. 1: Safe Prevention of the Primary Cesarean Delivery." *Obstetrics &*

Gynecology, vol. 123, no. 3, 2014, pp. 693-711, https://10.1097/01. AOG.0000444441.04111.1d.

47 Tsvieli, O., et al. "Risk factors and perinatal outcome of pregnancies complicated with cephalopelvic disproportion: a population-based study." *Archives of Gynecology and Obstetrics,* vol. 285, 2012, pp. 931–936, https://doi.org/10.1007/s00404-011-2086-4.

48 Romero, Roberto. "A profile of Emanuel A. Friedman, MD." *American Journal of Obstetrics & Gynecology*, vol 215, no. 4, 2016, pp. 413 – 414, https://www.ajog.org/article/S0002-9378(16)30469-0/fulltext.

49 Pearson, Catherine. "The conventional wisdom on how long normal labor takes is all wrong." *HuffPost*, January 17, 2018, https://www.google.com/amp/s/m.huffpost.com/us/entry/us_5a5e4420e4b0c59bc1f94d38/amp.

50 Eri, Tine, et al. "'Stay home for as long as possible': Midwives' priorities and strategies in communicating with first-time mothers in early labour." *Midwifery,* vol. 27, no. 6, 2011, pp. 286-292. https://www.sciencedirect.com/science/article/abs/pii/S0266613811000088.

51 Lothian, Judith A. "Healthy birth practice #4: avoid interventions unless they are medically necessary." *The Journal of Perinatal Education,* vol. 23, no. 4, 2014, pp. 198-206, https://10.1891/1058-1243.23.4.198.

52 Jansen, Lauren, et al. "First Do No Harm: Interventions During Childbirth." *The Journal of Perinatal Education,* vol. 22, no. 2, 2013, pp. 83-92, https://10.1891/1058-1243.22.2.83.

53 World Health Organization. "WHO recommendation on intermittent fetal heart rate auscultation during labour." *The WHO Reproductive Health Library*, February 17, 2018, https://extranet. who.int/rhl/topics/preconception.

54 Lothian, Judith A. "Safe, Healthy Birth: What Every Pregnant Woman Needs to Know." *The Journal of Perinatal Education*, vol. 18, no. 3, 2009, pp. 48-54, https:10.1624/105812409X461225.

55 Dekker, Rebecca, and Anna Bertone. "The Evidence on: Fetal Monitoring." *Evidence Based Birth*, July 17, https://evidencebasedbirth.com/fetal-monitoring/.

56 Buttigieg, George, and Vella Massimo. "Neonatal Hypoxic Ischaemic Encephalopathy: Demolishing the Cerebral Palsy Myth and Enlightening Court Litigation." *Austin Pediatrics*, vol. 3, no. 4, 2016, pp. 1044.

57 Sartwelle, Thomas P., and James C. Johnston. "Continuous Electronic Fetal Monitoring during Labor: A Critique and a Reply to Contemporary Proponents." *Surgery Journal* (New York, N.Y.) vol. 4, no. 1, 2018, pp. e23-e28, https://10.1055/s-0038-1632404.

58 Clark, Steven L., and Gary D.V, Hankins. "Temporal and demographic trends in cerebral palsy- fact and fiction." *American Journal of Obstetrics and Gynecology*, March 1, 2003. https://doi.org/10.1067/mob.2003.204.

59 Bryant, Allison S., and Ann E. Borders. "Approaches to Limit Intervention During Labor and Birth." *American College of Obstetricians and Gynecologists*, February 2019, pp. 164–73, https://www.acog.org/clinical/clinical-guidance/committee-opinion/articles/2019/02/approaches-to-limit-intervention-during-labor-and-birth.

60 National Institute for Health and Care Excellence (NICE). "Intrapartum care for healthy women and babies." *Clinical guidelines,* December 3, 2014, updated February 21, 2017, https://www.nice.org.uk/guidance/cg190/chapter/Recommendations#monitoring-during-labour.

61 Goer, Henci. *"Epidurals: Do They or Don't They Increase Cesareans?."* The Journal of perinatal education vol. 24, no. 4, 2015, pp. 209-212, doi:10.1891/1058-1243.24.4.209

62 Warland, Jane. "Back to basics: avoiding the supine position in pregnancy." *The Journal of Physiology,* vol. 595, no. 4, 2017, pp. 1017-1018, https://www.ncbi.nlm.nih.gov/pmc/articles/PMC5309362/.

63 Sartwelle, Thomas P. "Electronic Fetal Monitoring: A Defense Lawyer's View." *Reviews in Obstetrics & Gynecology* vol. 5, no. 3-4, 2012, pp. e121-5.

64 Graham, Ernest, et al. "Diagnostic Accuracy of Fetal Heart Rate Monitoring in the Identification of Neonatal Encephalopathy." *Obstetrics & Gynecology,* vol. 124, no. 3, 2014, pp. 507-513, https://10.1097/AOG.0000000000000424.

65 "Fetal Heart Rate Monitoring Fails to Detect Brain Injury, Study Finds." *Johns Hopkins Medicine,* October 9, 2014. https://www.hopkinsmedicine.org/news/media/releases/fetal_heart_rate_monitoring_fails_to_detect_brain_injury_study_finds.

66 Grytten, J., et al. "Does the Use of Diagnostic Technology Reduce Fetal Mortality?" *Health Services Research,* vol. 53, 2018, pp. 4437-4459, https://10.1111/1475-6773.12721.

67 Han-Yang, Chen, et al. "Electronic Fetal Heart Rate Monitoring and its Relationship to Neonatal and Infant Mortality in the United States." *American Journal of Obstetrics and Gynecology,* vol. 204, no. 491, 2014, pp. e1-10.

68 Heelan, Lisa. "Fetal monitoring: creating a culture of safety with informed choice." *The Journal of Perinatal Education,* vol. 22, no. 3, 2013, pp. 156-65, https://10.1891/1058-1243.22.3.156.

69 Alfirevic, Zarko, et al. "Continuous cardiotocography (CTG) as a form of electronic fetal monitoring (EFM) for fetal assessment

during labour." *Cochrane Systemic Review*, February 3, 2017, https://doi.org/10.1002/14651858.CD006066.pub3.

70 Tharp, Barry R. "Neonatal Seizures and Syndromes." *Epilepsia*, vol. 43, no. s3, June 27, 2002, pp. 2-10, https://doi.org/10.1046/j.1528-1157.43.s.3.11.x.

71 Dyson, Charlotte, et al. "Could routine cardiotocography reduce long term cognitive impairment?" *BMJ (Clinical research ed.)*, vol. 342, 2012, pp. d3120, https://10.1136/bmj.d3120.

72 World Health Organization. "WHO recommendation on continuous cardiotography during labour." *The WHO Reproductive Health Library*, February 15, 2018, https://extranet.who.int/rhl/topics/preconception-pregnancy-childbirth-and-postpartum-care/care-during-childbirth/care-during-labour-1st-stage/who-recommendation-continuous-cardiotocography-during-labour.

73 World Health Organization. "WHO recommendation on intermittent fetal heart rate auscultation during labour." *The WHO Reproductive Health Library*, February 17, 2018, https://extranet.who.int/rhl/topics/preconception.

74 Levy, D. M. "FRCA, Pre-operative fasting—60 years on from Mendelson, Continuing Education." *Anaesthesia Critical Care & Pain*, volume 6, no. 6, December 2006, pp. 215–218, https://doi.org/10.1093/bjaceaccp/mkl048.

75 Knott, Laurence. "Mendelson's Syndrome." *Patient Access*, vol. 1284, no. 23, February 1, 2015, https://medical.azureedge.net/pdf/1284.pdf?v=636700479176315654; https://patient.info/doctor/mendelsons-syndrome.

76 Sleutel, M., and S. S. Golden. "Fasting in labor: relic or requirement." *Journal of Obstetric, Gynecologic, and Neonatal Nursing*, vol. 28, no. 5, 1999, pp. 507-12, https:10.1111/j.1552-6909.1999.tb02024.x.

77 "Most healthy women would benefit from light meal during labor." *American Society of Anesthesiologists*, November 6, 2015, https://www.asahq.org/about-asa/newsroom/news-releases/2015/11/eating-a-light-meal-during-labor.

78 Al-Dossari, Rabhah, et al. "Effect of eating dates and drinking water versus IV fluids during labor on labor and neonatal outcomes." *IOSR Journal of Nursing and Health Science*, ver. III, volume 6, no. 4, July-August 2017, pp. 86-94, https://pdfs.semanticscholar.org/8621/bbe00b02c88014b862f86e9747ef4745a31c.pdf.

79 Sperling, Jeffrey D., et al. "Restriction of oral intake during labor: whither are we bound?" *American Journal of Obstetrics and Gynecology*, vol. 214, no. 5, 2016, pp. 592-6, https://10.1016/j.ajog.2016.01.166.

80 Chantry, Caroline J. "Excess Weight Loss in First-Born Breastfed Newborns Relates to Maternal Intrapartum Fluid Balance." *Pediatrics*, vol. 127, no. 1, 2011, pp. e171-e179, https://doi.org/10.1542/peds.2009-2663.

81 Tita, Alan T.N., and William W. Andrews. "Diagnosis and management of clinical chorioamnionitis." *Clinics in Perinatology*, vol. 37, no. 2, 2010, pp. 339-54, https://10.1016/j.clp.2010.02.003.

82 Ahmed, Waleed A.S., and Mostafa Ahmed Hamdy. "Optimal management of umbilical cord prolapse." *International Journal of Womens Health*, vol. 10, 2018, pp. 459-465, https://doi.org/10.2147/IJWH.S130879.

83 Kawakita, T., et al. "Risk Factors for Umbilical Cord Prolapse at the Time of Artificial Rupture of Membranes." *American Journal of Perinatology Reports*, vol. 8, 2018, pp. e89–e94, https://www.thieme-connect.de/products/ejournals/pdf/10.1055/s-0038-1649486.pdf.

84 Informed Health. "Pregnancy and birth: Epidurals and painkillers for labor pain relief." *Institute for Quality and Efficiency*

in Health Care, March 3, 2006, updated March 22, 2018, https://www.ncbi.nlm.nih.gov/books/NBK279567/?report=reader#_NBK279567_pubdet_.

85 Greenwell, Elizabeth A., et al. "Intrapartum Temperature Elevation, Epidural Use, and Adverse Outcome in Term Infants." *Pediatrics*, February 2012, 129 (2) e447-e454; DOI: https://doi.org/10.1542/peds.2010-2301.

86 Informed Health. "Pregnancy and birth: Epidurals and painkillers for labor pain relief." *Institute for Quality and Efficiency in Health Care*, March 3, 2006, updated March 22, 2018, https://www.ncbi.nlm.nih.gov/books/NBK279567/?report=reader#_NBK279567_pubdet_.

87 Informed Health. "Pregnancy and birth: Epidurals and painkillers for labor pain relief." *Institute for Quality and Efficiency in Health Care*, March 3, 2006, updated March 22, 2018, https://www.ncbi.nlm.nih.gov/books/NBK279567/?report=reader#_NBK279567_pubdet_.

88 Ballantyne, J.C., et al. "Itching after epidural and spinal opiates." *Pain*, vol. 33, no. 2, 1988, pp. 149-60, https://10.1016/0304-3959(88)90085-1.

89 Ghaleb, Ahmed. "Postdural Puncture Headache." *Anesthesiology Research and Practice,* vol. 2010, (2010): 102967, https://10.1155/2010/102967.

90 Gurudatt, C. L. "Unintentional dural puncture and postdural puncture headache-can this headache of the patient as well as the anaesthesiologist be prevented?" *Indian Journal of Anaesthesia,* vol. 58, no. 4, 2014, pp. 385-7, https://10.4103/0019-5049.138962.

91 Dekker, Rebecca. "Effects of Epidurals on the Second Stage of Labor." *Evidence Based Birth,* 2018, https://evidencebasedbirth.com/effects-of-epidurals-on-the-second-stage-of-labor/.

92 Cheng, Yvonne W., et al. "Second Stage of Labor and Epidural Use: A Larger Effect Than Previously Suggested." *Obstetrics & Gynecology,* vol. 123, no. 3, 2014, pp. 527-535, hyyps://10.1097/AOG.0000000000000134.

93 "Assisted Vaginal Delivery." *ACOG,* February 2016, https://www.acog.org/patient-resources/faqs/labor-delivery-and-postpartum-care/assisted-vaginal-delivery.

94 Dekker, Rebecca. "Evidence on: Prolonged Second Stage of Labor". *Evidence Based Birth,* May 24, 2017.

95 Belghiti, Jérémie, et al. "Oxytocin during labour and risk of severe postpartum haemorrhage: a population-based, cohort-nested case-control study." *BMJ Open,* vol. 1, no. 2, 2011, pp. e000514, https://10.1136/bmjopen-2011-000514.

96 Memon, Hafsa U. and Victoria L. Handa. "Vaginal childbirth and pelvic floor disorders." *Women's Health,* vol. 9, no. 3, 2013, pp. 265-77, https://10.2217/whe.13.17.

97 Fitzgerald, Mary P. et al. "Risk factors for anal sphincter tear during vaginal delivery." *Obstetrics and Gynecology,* vol. 109, no. 1, 2007, pp. 29-34. https://10.1097/01.AOG.0000242616.56617.ff.

98 Cheng, Yvonne W., et al. "Timing of operative vaginal delivery and associated perinatal outcomes in nulliparous women." *The Journal of Maternal-Fetal & Neonatal Medicine,* vol. 24, no. 5, 2011, pp. 692-697, https://10.3109/14767058.2010.521872.

99 Elvander, Charlotte, et al. "Birth position and obstetric anal sphincter injury: a population-based study of 113 000 spontaneous births." *BMC Pregnancy and Childbirth,* vol. 15, 2015, pp. 252, https://10.1186/s12884-015-0689-7.

100 Roberts, Christine L., et al. "A meta-analysis of upright positions in the second stage to reduce instrumental deliveries in women with epidural analgesia." *Acta Obstetricia et Gynecologica*

Scandinavica, vol. 84, no. 8, 2005, pp. 794-8, https://10.1111/j.0001-6349.2005.00786.x.

101 Dekker, Rebecca. "The Evidence on: Birthing Positions." *Evidence Based Birth,* October 2, 2012, updated February 2, 2018, https://evidencebasedbirth.com/evidence-birthing-positions/.

102 Watson, Helen L., and Alison Cooke. "What influences women's movement and the use of different positions during labour and birth: a systematic review protocol." *Systemic Reviews,* vol. 188, 2018, https://doi.org/10.1186/s13643-018-0857-8.

103 Ahmadi, Zohre, et al. "Effect of Breathing Technique of Blowing on the Extent of Damage to the Perineum at the Moment of Delivery: A Randomized Clinical Trial." *Iranian Journal of Nursing and Midwifery Research,* vol. 22, no. 1, 2017, pp. 62-66, https://10.4103/1735-9066.202071.

104 Simpson, Kathleen Rice, and Dotti C. James. "Effects of Immediate Versus Delayed Pushing During Second-Stage Labor on Fetal Well-Being: A Randomized Clinical Trial." *Nursing Research,* vol. 54, no. 3, 2005, pp. 149-157, https://journals.lww.com/nursingresearchonline/Abstract/2005/05000/Effects_of_Immediate_Versus_Delayed_Pushing_During.2.aspx.

105 Ahmadi, Zohre, et al. "Effect of Breathing Technique of Blowing on the Extent of Damage to the Perineum at the Moment of Delivery: A Randomized Clinical Trial." *Iranian Journal of Nursing and Midwifery Research,* vol. 22, no. 1, 2017, pp. 62-66. https://10.4103/1735-9066.202071.

106 Brancato, Robyn M., et al. "A meta-analysis of passive descent versus immediate pushing in nulliparous women with epidural analgesia in the second stage of labor." *JOGNN,* vol. 37, no. 4-12, 2008, https://10.1111/j.1552-6909.2007.00205.x https://www.jognn.org/article/S0884-2175(15)33722-9/pdf.

107 Fraser, W.D. et al. "Multicenter, randomized, controlled trial of delayed pushing for nulliparous women in the second stage of labor with continuous epidural analgesia. The PEOPLE (Pushing Early or Pushing Late with Epidural) Study Group." *American Journal of Obstetrics and Gynecology,* vol. 182, no. 5, 2000, pp. 1165-72, https://10.1067/mob.2000.105197.

108 Simpson, Kathleen Rice. "When and how to push: providing the most current information about second-stage labor to women during childbirth education." *The Journal of Perinatal Education,* vol. 15, no. 4, 2006, pp. 6-9, https://10.1624/105812406X151367.

109 Mayo Clinic Staff. "Episiotomy: When it's needed, when it's not." *Mayo Clinic,* October 23, 2018, https://www.mayoclinic.org/healthy-lifestyle/labor-and-delivery/in-depth/episiotomy/art-20047282.

110 Jiang H., et al. "Selective versus routine use of episiotomy for vaginal birth." *Cochrane Database of Systematic Reviews,* no. 2, 2017, https://10.1002/14651858.CD000081.pub3.

111 Janssen, Patricia A., et al. "Outcomes of planned hospital birth attended by midwives compared with physicians in British Columbia." *Birth,* vol. 34, no. 2, 2007, pp. 140-147, https://10.1111/j.1523-536X.2007.00160.x.

112 Sandall, Jane, et al. "Midwife-led continuity models versus other models of care for childbearing women." *Cochrane Database of Systematic Reviews,* April 28, 2016, https://doi.org/10.1002/14651858.CD004667.pub5.

113 Kuiper, Renske. "Interview with Renske Kuiper, Dutch Home midwife." *Home Birth Mom,* 2018, http://homebirthmom.com/interview-with-renske-kuiper-dutch-homebirth-midwife/.

114 Cobell, Anne. "Interview with Anne Cobell, British midwife." *Home Birth Mom,* 2018, http://homebirthmom.com/interview-with-anne-cobell-british-midwife/.

115 Dahlen, Hannah. "Interview with Professor Hannah Dahlen, Australian Home Birth Midwife." *Home Birth Mom,* 2019, http://homebirthmom.com/interview-with-professor-hannah-dahlen-australian-home-birth-midwife/.

116 Engel, Yetty. "Interview with Mrs. Yetty Engel, CM." *Home Birth Mom,* 2018, http://homebirthmom.com/yetty-engel-homebirth-midwife/.

117 Lamar, Michael, et al. "Jelly beans as an alternative to a fifty-gram glucose beverage for gestational diabetes screening." *American Journal of Obstetrics and Gynecology,* vol. 181, no. 5, 1999, http://citeseerx.ist.psu.edu/viewdoc/download?doi=10.1.1.1048.1031&rep=rep1&type=pdf.

118 Heath, Chip, and Dan Heath. *The Power of Moments.* Simon and Schuster, 2017.

119 Aune, Ingvild, et al. "Nature works best when allowed to run its course. The experience of midwives promoting normal births in a home birth setting." *Midwifery,* vol. 50, 2017, pp. 21-26, https://10.1016/j.midw.2017.03.020.

120 Griffin, Jennifer. "Jennifer Griffin: A home birth story." *Home Birth Mom,* 2018, http://homebirthmom.com/jennifer-griffin-homebirth-story/.

121 Griffin, Jennifer. *Understanding Morning Sickness As A Gift: An Introspective Story of Healing and Hope from a Hyperemesis Gravidarum Survivor.* E-book, Spiritual Gift Institute, 2018, https://www.amazon.com/Understanding-Morning-Sickness-Gift-Introspective-ebook/dp/B076MLS29T.

122 Cole, Jessica. "Jessica Cole: A home birth story." *Home Birth Mom,* 2017, http://homebirthmom.com/jessica-cole-homebirth-story/.

123 Van Haaren- Ten Haken, Tamar. "Interview with Tamar Van Haaren-Ten Haken, professor and home birth midwife." *Home*

Birth Mom, 2019, http://homebirthmom.com/interview-with-tamar-van-haaren-ten-haken-professor-and-home-birth-midwife/.

124 Kuiper, Renske. "Interview with Renske Kuiper, Dutch Home midwife." *Home Birth Mom,* 2018, http://homebirthmom.com/interview-with-renske-kuiper-dutch-homebirth-midwife/.

125 Engel, Yetty. "Interview with Mrs. Yetty Engel, CM." *Home Birth Mom,* 2018, http://homebirthmom.com/yetty-engel-homebirth-midwife/.

126 "State by State." *Midwives Alliance of North America,* 2020, https://mana.org/about-midwives/state-by-state.

127 "How to become a CPM". *NARM,* 2020, https://narm.org/certification/how-to-become-a-cpm/.

128 *North American Registry of Midwives.* NARM, 1992-2020, http://narm.org.

129 "CNM, CPM, CM, Doula: Understanding Midwifery Roles, Credentials, and Scope of Practice." *Midwifeschooling.com,* 2020, https://www.midwifeschooling.com/midwifery-roles-and-credentials/.

130 "The Credential CNM and CM." *American College of Nurse Midwives,* 2020, https://www.midwife.org/The-Credential-CNM-and-CM.

131 Ben Natan, Merav, and Mally Ehrenfeld. "Nursing and midwifery education, practice, and issues in Israel." *Nursing & Health Sciences,* vol. 13, no. 1-3, 2011, https://10.1111/j.1442-2018.2011.00582.x.

132 Ben Ami, Barbara. "Interview with Barbara Ben Ami, a home birth midwife in Israel." *Home Birth Mom,* 2018, http://homebirthmom.com/interview-with-barbara-ben-ami-a-homebirth-midwife-in-israel/.

133 Ben Ami, Barbara. "About." *Home Birth Israel,* 2020, https://www.homebirthisrael.com/en/about/.

134 Dahlen, Hannah. "Interview with Professor Hannah Dahlen, Australian Home Birth Midwife." *Home Birth Mom,* 2019, http://homebirthmom.com/interview-with-professor-hannah-dahlen-australian-home-birth-midwife/.

135 Jacobs, Chaya. "Chaya Jacobs: A home birth story." *Home Birth Mom,* 2018, http://homebirthmom.com/chaya-jacobs-a-homebirth-story/.

136 Dekker, Rebecca, and Anna Bertone. "Evidence on: The Vitamin K Shot in Newborns." *Evidence Based Birth*, March 18, 2014, updated April 9, 2019, https://evidencebasedbirth.com/evidence-for-the-vitamin-k-shot-in-newborns/.

137 Dekker, Rebecca, and Anna Bertone. "The Evidence on: Erythromycin Eye Ointment for Newborns." *Evidence Based Birth*. Published November 12, 2012, updated November 6, 2019, https://evidencebasedbirth.com/is-erythromycin-eye-ointment-always-necessary-for-newborns/.

138 Marinelli, Leah. "Interview with Home Birth Midwife Leah Marinelli." *Home Birth Mom,* 2018, http://homebirthmom.com/interview-with-homebirth-midwife-leah-marinelli/.

139 Dekker, Rebecca. "The Evidence on: Waterbirth." *Evidence Based Birth*, July 8, 2014, updated on January 30, 2018, https://evidencebasedbirth.com/waterbirth/.

140 Geissbuehler, Verena, et al. "Waterbirths compared with landbirths: an observational study of nine years." *Journal of Perinatal Medicine,* vol. 32, no.4, 2004, pp. 308 314, https://10.1515/JPM.2004.057.

141 Chaichian, Shahla, et al. "Experience of water birth delivery in Iran." *Archives of Iranian Medicine,* vol. 12, no. 5, 2009, pp. 468 471.

142 "Water Labor and Water Birth." *International Childbirth Education Association*, October 2015, https://icea.org/wp-content/uploads/2016/01/Water_Birth_PP.pdf.

143 "The 'Whole-istic' DIAH Home Birth Preparation Checklist." *Doing It At Home: Our Home Birth Podcast*, from DIAH, April 29, 2018, https://www.diahpodcast.com/single-post/The-Home-Birth-Preparation-Checklist.

144 Simavli, Serap, et al. "Effect of Music on Labor Pain Relief, Anxiety Level and Postpartum Analgesic Requirement: A Randomized Controlled Clinical Trial." *Gynecologic and Obstetric Investigation,* vol. 78, 2014, https://10.1159/000365085.

145 *Hypnobirthing International, The Mongan Method.* Hypnobirthing, 2020, https://us.hypnobirthing.com.

146 Lewis, Sarah. "Sarah Lewis: A home birth story." *Home Birth Mom,* 2017, http://homebirthmom.com/sarah-lewis-homebirth-story/.

147 "The Role of Hormones in Childbirth." *Childbirth Connection,* 2020, http://www.childbirthconnection.org/maternity-care/role-of-hormones/.

148 Buckley, Sarah. "Undisturbed Birth." *AIMS Journal,* vol. 23, no. 4, 2011, https://www.aims.org.uk/journal/item/undisturbed-birth.

149 Ben Ami, Barbara. "Interview with Barbara Ben Ami, a home birth midwife in Israel." *Home Birth Mom,* 2018, http://homebirthmom.com/interview-with-barbara-ben-ami-a-homebirth-midwife-in-israel/.

150 Bohren, Meghan A., et al. "Continuous support for women during childbirth." *The Cochrane Database of Systematic Reviews,* vol. 7, no. 7, 2017, https://10.1002/14651858.CD003766.pub6.

151 The Bump Editors. "Writing a birth plan? There's a tool for that." *The Bump,* updated May 2017, https://www.thebump.com/a/tool-birth-plan/amp.

152 Pearlman, Ruthie. "Ruthie Pearlman: A home birth story." *Home Birth Mom,* 2017, http://homebirthmom.com/ruthie-pearlman-homebirth-story/.

153 Tully, Gail. "Roll-over." *Maternity House Publishing,* 2020, https://spinningbabies.com/learn-more/techniques/other-techniques/roll-over/.

154 "Chiropractic adjustment". *Mayo* Clinic, 2020, https://www.mayoclinic.org/tests-procedures/chiropractic-adjustment/about/pac-20393513.

155 Griffin, Jennifer. "Jennifer Griffin: A home birth story." *Home Birth Mom,* 2018, http://homebirthmom.com/jennifer-griffin-homebirth-story/.

156 Schlaeger, Judith M., et al. "Acupuncture and Acupressure in Labor." *Journal of Midwifery & Women's Health,* vol. 62, no. 1, 2017, pp. 12-28, https://10.1111/jmwh.12545.

157 Pohlner, Karen. "Acupressure for pain relief during labour." *Pregnancy Birth & Beyond,* 2020, https://www.pregnancy.com.au/acupressure-pain-relief-labour/.

158 Davis, April. "Interview with April Davis, home birth doula and EMT." *Home Birth Mom,* 2017, http://homebirthmom.com/interview-homebirth-doula-emt-april-davis/.

159 Lewis, Sarah. "Sarah Lewis: A home birth story." *Home Birth Mom,* 2017, http://homebirthmom.com/sarah-lewis-homebirth-story/.

160 Levy, Shoshana. "Shoshana Levy: a home birth story." *Home Birth Mom,* 2017, http://homebirthmom.com/shoshana-levy-homebirth-story/.

161 Marinelli, Leah. "Interview with Home Birth Midwife Leah Marinelli." *Home Birth Mom,* 2018, http://homebirthmom.com/interview-with-homebirth-midwife-leah-marinelli/.

162 Ahmed, Waleed A.S., and Mostafa Ahmed Hamdy. "Optimal management of umbilical cord prolapse." *International Journal of Women's Health,* vol. 10, 2018, pp. 459-465, https://10.2147/IJWH. S130879.

163 Hasegawa, Junichi, et al. "Obstetric risk factors for umbilical cord prolapse: a nationwide population-based study in Japan." *Archives of Gynecology and Obstetrics,* vol. 294, no. 3, 2016, pp. 467-72, https://10.1007/s00404-015-3996-3.

164 Ahmed, Waleed A.S., and Mostafa Ahmed Hamdy. "Optimal management of umbilical cord prolapse." *International Journal of Women's Health,* vol. 10, 2018, pp. 459-465, https://10.2147/IJWH. S130879.

165 McLintock, C., and A.H. James. "Obstetric hemorrhage." *Journal of Thrombosis and Haemostasis,* vol. 9, 2011, pp. 1441-1451, doi:10.1111/j.1538-7836.2011.04398.x.

166 Parikh, Reshma, et al. "Cervical lacerations: some surprising facts." *American Journal of Obstetrics and Gynecology,* vol. 196, no. 5, 2007, pp. e17–18, doi: 10.1016/j.ajog.2006.11.043.

167 Nove, Andrea, et al. "Comparing the odds of postpartum haemorrhage in planned home birth against planned hospital birth: results of an observational study of over 500,000 maternities in the UK." *BMC Pregnancy Childbirth,* vol. 12, no. 130, 2012, https:// doi.org/10.1186/1471-2393-12-130.

168 Khireddine, Imane et al. "Induction of labor and risk of postpartum hemorrhage in low risk parturients." *PloS One,* vol. 8, no. 1, 2013, pp. e54858, https://10.1371/journal.pone.0054858.

169 Tita, Alan T.N., and William W. Andrews. "Diagnosis and management of clinical chorioamnionitis." *Clinics in Perinatology,* vol. 37, no. 2, 2010, pp. 339-54, https://10.1016/j.clp.2010.02.003.

170 Vasa, Rohitkumar, et al. "Nuchal cord at delivery and perinatal outcomes: Single-center retrospective study, with emphasis on

fetal acid-base balance." *Pediatrics and Neonatology*, vol. 59, no. 5, 2018, pp. 439-447, https://10.1016/j.pedneo.2018.03.002.

171 Tikkanen, Minaa, et al. "Clinical presentation and risk factors of placental abruption." *Acta Obstetricia et Gynecologica Scandinavica*, vol. 85, no. 6, 2006, pp. 700-705, https://10.1080/00016340500449915.

172 Getahun, Darios, et al. "Previous Cesarean Delivery and Risks of Placenta Previa and Placental Abruption." *Obstetrics and Gynecology*, vol. 107, no. 4, 2006, pp. 771-778, https://10.1097/01. AOG.0000206182.63788.80.

173 Tikkanen, Minna. "Placental abruption: epidemiology, risk factors and consequences." *Acta Obstetricia et Gynecologica Scandinavica*, vol. 90, no. 2, 2011, pp. 140-9, https://10.1111/j.1600-0412.2010.01030.x.

174 Raju, U., et al. "Meconium Aspiration Syndrome: An Insight." *Medical Journal, Armed Forces India,* vol. 66, no. 2, 2010, pp. 152-7, https://10.1016/S0377-1237(10)80131-5.

175 Kumari, Rekha et al. "Foetal outcome in patients with meconium stained liquor." *JPMA The Journal of the Pakistan Medical Association*, vol. 62, no. 5, 2012, pp. 474-6.

176 "What is Amniotic Fluid Embolism?" *AFE Foundation*, 2018, https://www.afesupport.org/what-is-amniotic-fluid-embolism/#1447098231154-78c0b784-7247.

177 Knight, Marian, et al. "Incidence and risk factors for amniotic-fluid embolism." *Obstetrics and Gynecology*, vol. 115, no. 5, 2010, pp. 910-7, https://10.1097/AOG.0b013e3181d9f629.

178 Rattray, Darrien D., et al. "Acute disseminated intravascular coagulation in obstetrics: a tertiary centre population review (1980 to 2009)." *Journal of Obstetrics and Gynaecology Canada, JOGC = Journal D'obstetrique et Gynecologie du Canada*: JOGC, vol. 34, no. 4, 2012, pp. 341-347, https://10.1016/s1701-2163(16)35214-8.

179 The World Bank Data. "Maternal mortality ratio." *World Health Organization*, 2019, https://data.worldbank.org/indicator/SH.STA.MMRT?locations=FI-VE&name_desc=true&year_high_desc=false.

180 Kuiper, Renske. "Interview with Renske Kuiper, Dutch Home midwife." *Home Birth Mom*, 2018, http://homebirthmom.com/interview-with-renske-kuiper-dutch-homebirth-midwife/.

181 Primavesi, Carina. "Carina Primavesi: A home birth story in Holland." *Home Birth Mom*, 2018, http://homebirthmom.com/carina-primavesi-homebirth-story-holland/.

182 De Jonge, Ank. "Interview with Ank de Jonge. Dutch home birth researcher." *Home Birth Mom*, 2018, http://homebirthmom.com/interview-ank-de-jonge-homebirth-midwife-researcher/.

183 Van Haaren-ten Haken, T. M. "The Place To Be: Women's birth place preferences in the Netherlands." *Maastricht University*, 2018, https://doi.org/10.26481/dis.20180518th.

184 Evers, Annemieke C.C., et al. "Perinatal mortality and severe morbidity in low and high risk term pregnancies in the Netherlands: prospective cohort study." *BMJ (Clinical research ed.),* vol. 341, 2010, pp. c5639, https://10.1136/bmj.c5639.

185 Van Haaren-Ten Haken, Tamar. "Interview with Tamar Van Haaren-Ten Haken, professor and home birth midwife." *Home Birth Mom*, 2019, http://homebirthmom.com/interview-with-tamar-van-haaren-ten-haken-professor-and-home-birth-midwife/.

186 Van Haaren-ten Haken, T. M. "The Place To Be: Women's birth place preferences in the Netherlands." *Maastricht University*, 2018, https://doi.org/10.26481/dis.20180518th.

187 de Jonge, A., et al. "Perinatal mortality and morbidity up to 28 days after birth among 743 070 low-risk planned home and hospital births: a cohort study based on three merged national perinatal

databases." *BJOG : an international journal of obstetrics and gynaecology*, vol. 122, no. 5, 2015, pp. 720-8, https://10.1111/1471-0.

188 de Jonge, Ank. "Interview with Ank de Jonge, Dutch home birth researcher." *Home Birth Mom*, 2018, http://homebirthmom. com/interview-ank-de-jonge-homebirth-midwife-researcher/.

189 Bazian. "Nice recommends home births for some mums." *NHS*, December 3, 2014, https://www.nhs.uk/news/pregnancy-and-child/nice-recommends-home-births-for-some-mums/.

190 Birthplace in England Collaborative Group, and P. Brocklehurt. "Perinatal and maternal outcomes by planned place of birth for healthy women with low risk pregnancies: the Birthplace in England national prospective cohort study." *BMJ (Clinical research ed.)*, vol. 343, 2011, pp. d7400, https://10.1136/bmj.d7400.

191 Janssen, Patricia A., et al. "Outcomes of planned home birth with registered midwife versus planned hospital birth with midwife or physician." *CMAJ : Canadian Medical Association Journal = Journal de l'Association Medicale Canadienne*, vol. 181, no. 6-7, 2009, pp. 377-83, https://10.1503/cmaj.081869.

192 Hutton, Eileen K., et al. "Outcomes associated with planned place of birth among women with low-risk pregnancies." *CMAJ : Canadian Medical Association Journal = Journal de l'Association Medicale Canadienne,* vol. 188, no. 5, 2016, pp. E80-E90, https://10.1503/cmaj.150564.

193 de Jonge, Ank. "Interview with Ank de Jonge, Dutch home birth researcher." *Home Birth Mom*, 2018, http://homebirthmom. com/interview-ank-de-jonge-homebirth-midwife-researcher/.

194 de Jonge, A., et al. "Perinatal mortality and morbidity up to 28 days after birth among 743 070 low-risk planned home and hospital births: a cohort study based on three merged national perinatal databases." *BJOG : an international journal of obstetrics and gynaecology*, vol. 122, no. 5, 2015, pp. 720-8.

195 Snowden, Jonathan M., et al. "Planned Out-of-Hospital Birth and Birth Outcomes." *The New England Journal of Medicine*, vol. 373, no. 27, 2015, pp. 2642-53, https://10.1056/NEJMsa1501738.

196 Hart, Gail, and Judy Slome Cohain. "Midwifery Today Responds to Study Questioning Homebirth Safety." *Midwifery Today*, 2010. https://midwiferytoday.com/mt-articles/ajog-response/.

197 Wang, Amy. "Most Oregon births are safe, but home births are riskier for babies, OHSU says." *The Oregonian/Oregon Live*, December 30, 2015, updated January 9, 2019, https://www.oregonlive.com/health/2015/12/home_births_hospital_births.html.

198 Le Coz, Emily, et al. "Dodging punishment: How a burgeoning industry fails to hold midwives accountable." *The Daytona Beach News-Journal*, December 27, 2018, https://www.google.com/amp/s/www.news-journalonline.com/news/20181227/dodging-punishment-how-burgeoning-industry-fails-to-hold-midwives-accountable%3ftemplate=ampart.

199 Davis, April. "Interview with April Davis, home birth doula and EMT." *Home Birth Mom,* 2017, http://homebirthmom.com/interview-homebirth-doula-emt-april-davis/.

200 *Birth by the Numbers*, 2018, https://www.birthbythenumbers.org/

201 Declercq, Eugene. "Interview with Eugene Declercq." *Home Birth Mom,* 2019, http://homebirthmom.com/interview-with-eugene-declercq/.

202 Caughey, Aaron B., and Melissa Cheyney. "Home and Birth Center Birth in the United States: Time for Greater Collaboration Across Models of Care." *Obstetrics and Gynecology,* vol. 133, no. 5, 2019, pp. 1033-1050, https://10.1097/AOG.0000000000003215.

203 Dahlen, Hannah. "Interview with Professor Hannah Dahlen, Australian Home Birth Midwife." *Home Birth Mom*, 2019, http://

homebirthmom.com/interview-with-professor-hannah-dahlen-australian-home-birth-midwife/.

204 Dahlen, Hannah, et al. *Birthing Outside the System: The Canary in the Coal Mine.* Routledge Research in Nursing and Midwifery, 2020.

205 Dahlen, Hannah. "Interview with Professor Hannah Dahlen, Australian Home Birth Midwife." *Home Birth Mom,* 2019, http:// homebirthmom.com/interview-with-professor-hannah-dahlen-australian-home-birth-midwife/.

206 Pascucci, Cristen. "Home birth versus hospital birth: you're missing the point, people." *Improving Birth,* February 17, 2014, https://improvingbirth.org/2014/02/versus/.

207 Dahlen, Hannah. "Interview with Professor Hannah Dahlen, Australian Home Birth Midwife." *Home Birth Mom,* 2019, http:// homebirthmom.com/interview-with-professor-hannah-dahlen-australian-home-birth-midwife/.

208 Scarf, Vanessa L., et al. "Maternal and perinatal outcomes by planned place of birth among women with low-risk pregnancies in high-income countries: A systematic review and meta-analysis." *Midwifery*, vol. 62, 2018, pp. 240-255, https://10.1016/j. midw.2018.03.024.

209 Committee on Obstetric Practice. "Committee Opinion No. 697: Planned Home Birth." *Obstetrics and Gynecology*, vol. 129, no. 4, 2017, pp. e117-e122, https://www.acog.org/clinical/clinical-guidance/committee-opinion/articles/2017/04/planned-home-birth.

210 "Global standards for midwifery education (2010)." *International Confederation of Midwives*, 2013, https://www. internationalmidwives.org/assets/files/general-files/2018/04/ icm-standards-guidelines_ammended2013.pdf.

211 Declercq, Eugene, and Naomi E. Stotland. "Planned home birth." *UpToDate*, April 26, 2017, https://www.porod-doma.cz/wp-content/uploads/2018/08/Planned-home-birth-UpToDate.pdf.

212 "Planned Birth at Home in South Australia: Clinical Directive." *Government of South Australia*, 2018, https://www.sahealth.sa.gov.au/wps/wcm/connect/76aaf1004f3219c488eefd080fa6802e/Planned+Birth+at+Home+in+SA+2018_CD_v3_0.pdf?MOD=AJPERES&CACHEID=ROOTWORKSPACE-76aaf1004f3219c488eefd080fa6802e-mSV8hlX.

213 Pearlman, Ruthie. "Ruthie Pearlman: A home birth story." *Home Birth Mom,* 2017, http://homebirthmom.com/ruthie-pearlman-homebirth-story/.

214 Ben Ami, Barbara. "Interview with Barbara Ben Ami, a home birth midwife in Israel." *Home Birth Mom,* 2018, http://homebirthmom.com/interview-with-barbara-ben-ami-a-homebirth-midwife-in-israel/.

215 Hodnett, Ellen D. et al. "Continuous support for women during childbirth." *The Cochrane Database of Systematic Reviews,* vol. 7, 2013, pp. CD003766, https://10.1002/14651858.CD003766.pub5.

216 Kuiper, Renske. "Interview with Renske Kuiper, Dutch Home midwife." *Home Birth Mom,* 2018, http://homebirthmom.com/interview-with-renske-kuiper-dutch-homebirth-midwife/.

217 Lothian, Judith A. "Do not disturb: the importance of privacy in labor." *The Journal of Perinatal Education,* vol. 13, no. 3, 2004, pp. 4-6, https://10.1624/105812404X1707.

218 Scott, Elizabeth. "All About Catecholamines in the Stress Response." *Verywell mind*, updated July 27, 2020, https://www.verywellmind.com/all-about-catecholamines-3145098.

219 Wagner, Marsden. "Born in the USA: How a broken maternity system must be fixed to put women and children first." *University of California Press*, 2006, pp.177-181.

220 Davis, April. "Interview with April Davis, home birth doula and EMT." *Home Birth Mom*, 2017, http://homebirthmom.com/interview-homebirth-doula-emt-april-davis/.

221 Hodges, Susan. "Abuse in hospital-based birth settings?" *The Journal of Perinatal Education,* vol. 18, no. 4, 2009, pp. 8-11, doi:10.1624/105812409X474663.

222 Tucker, S. "There is a hidden epidemic of doctors abusing women in labor, doulas say". *Vice,* May 8, 2018, https://www.vice.com/amp/en_us/article/evqew7/obstetric-violence-doulas-abuse-giving-birth.

223 "Obstetric Violence." *Birth Monopoly,* 2020, https://birthmonopoly.com/obstetric-violence/.

224 Wagner, M. "Fish can't see water: the need to humanize birth." *International Journal of Gynaecology and Obstetrics*, vol. 75, 2001, pp. S25-37.

225 Reed, Rachel, et al. "Women's descriptions of childbirth trauma relating to care provider actions and interactions." *BMC Pregnancy and Childbirth,* vol. 17, no. 1, 2017, pp. 21, https://10.1186/s12884-016-1197-0.

226 Garthus-Niegel, Susan, et al. "The Impact of Postpartum Posttraumatic Stress and Depression Symptoms on Couples' Relationship Satisfaction: A Population-Based Prospective Study." *Frontiers in Psychology,* vol. 9, no. 1728, 2018, pp. 19, https://10.3389/fpsyg.2018.01728.

227 Pascucci, Cristen. "Nurses: women are not fabricating birth trauma." *Birth Monopoly,* November 4, 2015, https://birthmonopoly.com/nurses.

228 Garthus-Niegel, Susan, et al. "The Impact of Postpartum Posttraumatic Stress and Depression Symptoms on Couples' Relationship Satisfaction: A Population-Based Prospective Study." *Frontiers in Psychology*, vol. 9, no. 1728, 2018, pp. 19, https://10.3389/fpsyg.2018.01728.

229 Reed, Rachel, et al. "Women's descriptions of childbirth trauma relating to care provider actions and interactions." *BMC Pregnancy and Childbirth,* vol. 17, no. 1, 2017, pp. 21, https://10.1186/s12884-016-1197-0.

230 Modarres, Maryam, et al. "Prevalence and risk factors of childbirth-related post-traumatic stress symptoms." *BMC Pregnancy and Childbirth,* vol. 12, 2012, pp. 8, https://10.1186/1471-2393-12-88.

231 Reed, Rachel, et al. "Women's descriptions of childbirth trauma relating to care provider actions and interactions." *BMC Pregnancy and Childbirth,* vol. 17, no. 1, 2017, pp. 21, https://10.1186/s12884-016-1197-0.

232 Bosquet Enlow, Michelle, et al. "Maternal posttraumatic stress symptoms and infant emotional reactivity and emotion regulation." *Infant Behavior & Development,* vol. 34, no. 4, 2011, pp. 487-503, https://10.1016/j.infbeh.2011.07.007.

233 Rochaun, A. "Team birth project is proof that communication improves birth outcomes." *Scary Mommy,* December 18, 2018, https://www.scarymommy.com/team-birth-project/.

234 Schorow, Stephanie. "Media roundup: Team Birth Project gains national attention." *Ariadne Labs,* https://www.ariadnelabs.org/resources/articles/news/media-roundup-team-birth-project-gains-national-attention/. Accessed

235 Bebinger, Martha. "One twin's difficult birth puts a project designed to reduce c-sections to the test." *Kaiser Health News,* November 27, 2018, https://khn.org/news/reducing-cesarean-sections-even-for-difficult-deliveries/

236 Dekker, Rebecca. *Evidence Based Birth*, 2018, https://evidencebasedbirth. com.

237 McDonald, Susan J., et al. *"Effect of timing of umbilical cord clamping of term infants on maternal and neonatal outcomes."* Evidence-based Child Health: a Cochrane Review journal, vol. 9, no. 2, 2014, pp. 303-97, https://10.1002/ ebch.1971.

238 Mascola, Maria A., et al. "Delayed umbilical cord clamping after birth. Committee opinion no. 684." *American College of Obstetricians and Gynecologists,* January 2017, https://www.acog.org/clinical/clinical-guidance/committee-opinion/articles/2017/01/delayed-umbilical-cord-clamping-after-birth.

239 World Health Orginization. "Guideline: Delayed umbilical cord clamping for improved maternal and infant health and nutrition outcomes." *Geneva: World Health Organization,* 2014, https://apps. who.int/iris/bitstream/handle/10665/148793/9789241508209_eng. pdf;jsessionid=335A3EE5753196875B525D832CDC2A0C?sequence=1.

240 World Health Organization. "WHO recommendation on skin-to-skin contact.", *The WHO Reproductive Health Library*, February 17, 2018, https:// extranet.who.int/rhl/topics/newborn-health/care-newborn-infant/who-recommendation-skin-skin-contact-during-first-hour-after-birth.

241 Crenshaw, Jeannette T. "Healthy Birth Practice #6: Keep Mother and Baby Together- It's Best for Mother, Baby, and Breastfeeding." *The Journal of Perinatal Education,* vol. 23, no.4, 2014, pp. 211-7, htt ps://10.1891/1058-1243.23.4.211.

242 Bigelow, Ann, et al. "Effect of mother/infant skin-to-skin contact on postpartum depressive symptoms and maternal physiological stress." *Journal of Obstetric, Gynecologic, and Neonatal Nursing: JOGNN,* vol. 41, no. 3, 2012, pp. 369-82, https://10.1111/j.1552-6909.2012.01350.x.

243 Casas, Gloria. "Sherman nurse's 'wait to bathe' newborns policy adopted by hospitals." *Elgin Courier- News,* June 11, 2017, https://www.

chicagotribune.com/suburbs/elgin-courier-news/ct-ecn-elgin-sherman-nurse-baby-policy-st-0612-20170611-story.html.

244 Nishijima, Koji, et al. "Biology of the vernix caseosa: A review." *The Journal of Obstetrics and Gynaecology Research,* vol. 45, no. 11, 2019, pp. 2145-2149, https://10.1111/jog.14103.

245 Akinbi, Henry T., et al. "Host defense proteins in vernix caseosa and amniotic fluid." *American Journal of Obstetrics and Gynecology,* vol. 191, no. 6, 2004, pp. 2090-6, https://10.1016/j.ajog.2004.05.002.

246 Dekker, Rebecca. "Evidence confirms birth centers provide top-notch care." *American Association of Birth Centers,* January 31, 2013, https://www.birthcenters.org/page/NBCSII?.

247 Duke, Annie. *Thinking in Bets: Making Smarter Decisions When You Don't Have All the Facts.* Penguin Random House LLC, 2018.

248 *Hypnobirthing International, The Mongan Method.* Hypnobirthing, 2020, https://us.hypnobirthing.com.

249 "Childbirth Class." *Evidence Based Birth,* 2018, https://evidencebasedbirth.com/childbirth-class/.

250 Duke, Annie. *Thinking in Bets: Making Smarter Decisions When You Don't Have All the Facts.* Penguin Random House LLC, 2018, pp. 224.

251 Creedy, D., et al. "Birth trauma and post-traumatic stress disorder." *O&G magazine,* vol. 20, no. 3, Spring 2018, https://www.ogmagazine.org.au/20/3-20/birth-trauma-and-post-traumatic-stress-disorder-ptsd/.

252 Debrova, Yehudit. "Yehudit Debrova: A home birth story." *Home Birth Mom,* 2017, http://homebirthmom.com/yehudit-debrova-a-homebirth-story/.

253 Levy, Mindy. "Interview with Home Birth Midwife Mindy Levy." *Home Birth Mom,* 2018, http://homebirthmom.com/interview-with-homebirth-midwife-mindy-levy/.

254 Pearlman, Ruthie. "Ruthie Pearlman: A home birth story." *Home Birth Mom,* 2017, http://homebirthmom.com/ruthie-pearlman-homebirth-story/.

255 Davis, April. "Interview with April Davis, home birth doula and EMT." *Home Birth Mom,* 2017, http://homebirthmom.com/interview-homebirth-doula-emt-april-davis/.

256 Lewis, Sarah. "Sarah Lewis: A home birth story." *Home Birth Mom,* 2017, http://homebirthmom.com/sarah-lewis-homebirth-story/.

257 Griffin, Jennifer. "Jennifer Griffin: A home birth story." *Home Birth Mom,* 2018, http://homebirthmom.com/jennifer-griffin-homebirth-story/.

258 Marinelli, Leah. "Interview with Home Birth Midwife Leah Marinelli." *Home Birth Mom,* 2018, http://homebirthmom.com/interview-with-homebirth-midwife-leah-marinelli/.

259 Mongan, Marie. *HypnoBirthing: The Mongan method: A natural approach to a safe, easier, more comfortable birthing.* Health Communications, Inc., 2005.

www.ingramcontent.com/pod-product-compliance
Lightning Source LLC
Chambersburg PA
CBHW070838300326
41935CB00038B/1077